The PALEO BREAKFAST COOKBOOK

and Easy Gluten-Free Paleo Breakfast Recipes for a Paleo Diet

Rockridge Press

Copyright © 2013 by Rockridge Press, Berkeley, California

No part of this publication may be reproduced, stored in a retrieval system or transmitted in any form or by any means, electronic, mechanical, photocopying, recording, scanning or otherwise, except as permitted under Sections 107 or 108 of the 1976 United States Copyright Act, without the prior written permission of the Publisher. Requests to the Publisher for permission should be addressed to the Permissions Department, Rockridge Press, 918 Parker St, Suite A-12, Berkeley, CA 94710.

Limit of Liability/Disclaimer of Warranty: The Publisher and the author make no representations or warranties with respect to the accuracy or completeness of the contents of this work and specifically disclaim all warranties, including without limitation warranties of fitness for a particular purpose. No warranty may be created or extended by sales or promotional materials. The advice and strategies contained herein may not be suitable for every situation. This work is sold with the understanding that the publisher is not engaged in rendering medical, legal or other professional advice or services. If professional assistance is required, the services of a competent professional person should be sought. Neither the Publisher nor the author shall be liable for damages arising herefrom. The fact that an individual, organization or website is referred to in this work as a citation and/or potential source of further information does not mean that the author or the Publisher endorses the information the individual, organization or website may provide or recommendations they/it may make. Further, readers should be aware that Internet websites listed in this work may have changed or disappeared between when this work was written and when it is read.

For general information on our other products and services or to obtain technical support, please contact our Customer Care Department within the U.S. at (866) 744-2665, or outside the U.S. at (510) 253-0500.

Rockridge Press publishes its books in a variety of electronic and print formats. Some content that appears in print may not be available in electronic books, and vice versa.

TRADEMARKS: Rockridge Press and the Rockridge Press logo are trademarks or registered trademarks of Callisto Media Inc. and/or its affiliates, in the United States and other countries, and may not be used without written permission. All other trademarks are the property of their respective owners. Rockridge Press is not associated with any product or vendor mentioned in this book.

ISBN: Print 978-1-62315-136-2 | eBook 978-1-62315-135-5

CONTENTS

Introduction	1
Chapter 1: Why Eat a Paleo Breakfast?	2
Chapter 2: 10 Tips for Enjoying a Healthy Paleo Breakfast	4
Chapter 3: Paleo Slow Cooker Breakfasts	7
Steamed Hazelnut Breakfast Bread	7
Slow Cooker Almond Bread	9
Toasted Coconut Bread	10
Poached Pears with Cranberries	11
Dried Berry Compote	12
Cuban Pork and Plantain *Ropa Vieja*–Style Hash	13
Slow Cooker Pumpkin Butter	14
Vegetable Frittata	15
Sweet Potato and Chicken-Sausage Hash	16
Chapter 4: Paleo Shakes and Smoothies	17
Paleo Green Smoothie	17
Paleo Strawberry-Banana Smoothie	18
Protein Power Paleo Shake	19
Berrylicious Breakfast Smoothie	20

Tropical Island Shake ... 21
Nutty Carob Breakfast Smoothie ... 22
Green Power Morning Smoothie ... 23
Bright Day Citrus Smoothie ... 24
Key Lime Smoothie ... 25

Chapter 5: Paleo Breakfasts for Kids ... **26**

Waffles with Strawberry Compote ... 26
Banana Nut Pops ... 28
Yummy Paleo Granola ... 29
Egg and Sausage Muffins ... 30
Coconut-Pineapple Pancakes ... 31
Chocolate-Banana Breakfast Shake ... 32
Paleo Eggs Benedict ... 33
Eggs on Sweet Potato Rounds ... 34

Chapter 6: Paleo Breakfast Muffins ... **35**

Paleo Blueberry Muffins ... 35
Paleo "Bran" Muffins ... 37
"Oatmeal" Muffins ... 38
Apple Cranberry Breakfast Muffins ... 39
Bacon and Roasted Pepper Muffins ... 40
French Toast Muffins ... 41
Paleo Morning Glory Muffins ... 42
Chai Spiced Muffins ... 43

Chapter 7: Paleo Egg Breakfasts — 44

    Paleo Spinach Quiche — 44

    Paleo Frittata — 45

    Italian Scramble — 46

    Paleo Western Omelet — 47

    Paleo Egg White Omelet — 48

    Mushroom-Rosemary Omelet — 49

    Paleo Vegetable Omelet — 50

    Paleo Spinach Omelet — 51

    Paleo-Friendly Breakfast Egg Salad — 52

    Paleo Sausage Casserole — 53

Chapter 8: Paleo Pancakes and Waffles — 54

    Paleo Blueberry Pancakes — 54

    Paleo Coconut Flour Pancakes — 56

    Orange-Kissed Coconut Pancakes — 57

    Paleo Grain-Free Banana Pancakes — 58

    Mixed Berry Pancakes — 59

    Paleo Coconut Flour Waffles — 60

    Paleo Banana Waffles — 61

    Hazelnut Waffles — 62

Chapter 9: Paleo Eggless Breakfasts — 63

    Chicken-Wrapped Asparagus Spears with Pine Nut Mayo — 63

    Paleo Hash — 65

    Sautéed Chicken Livers — 66

Chicken and Mushroom Wraps　　　　　　　　　　　　67

　　　Paleo Sausage Gravy　　　　　　　　　　　　　　　68

　　　Toast with Mushroom Sauce　　　　　　　　　　　　69

　　　Paleo Crab Cakes　　　　　　　　　　　　　　　　70

　　　Sausage-Stuffed Portobello Mushrooms　　　　　　　71

　　　Turkey Steaks with Fried Apples　　　　　　　　　　72

Chapter 10: Paleo Breakfast Bars　　　　　　　　　　　　73

　　　Sweet Potato Breakfast Bars　　　　　　　　　　　　73

　　　Banana-Pecan Bars　　　　　　　　　　　　　　　　75

　　　Applesauce-Raisin Bars　　　　　　　　　　　　　　76

　　　Paleo Pumpkin Bars　　　　　　　　　　　　　　　77

　　　Fruity Coconut Bars　　　　　　　　　　　　　　　78

　　　Coconut-Almond Bars　　　　　　　　　　　　　　79

　　　Hazelnut-Peach Breakfast Bars　　　　　　　　　　　80

　　　Paleo Granola Bars　　　　　　　　　　　　　　　81

　　　No-Bake Fruit and Nut Bars　　　　　　　　　　　　82

Chapter 11: Living on the Paleo Diet　　　　　　　　　　83

Conclusion　　　　　　　　　　　　　　　　　　　　　99

Glossary　　　　　　　　　　　　　　　　　　　　　100

INTRODUCTION

With the enormous popularity of the Paleo diet, there's a real need for a wide variety of delicious, Paleo-friendly, gluten-free recipes. Any diet, no matter how healthy, can become monotonous if the same handful of meals is eaten week after week.

Breakfast is often the meal that falls into a rut the quickest. Because we're so busy, we tend to rely on just a few go-to meals or to skip breakfast altogether. This is a mistake, as a healthy breakfast is important for weight management, overall health, and the energy we need to get through the day.

In this book you'll find that a healthy and delicious Paleo and gluten-free breakfast doesn't take a lot of time or cost a lot to make. There are plenty of breakfasts that can be prepared ahead, such as the slow cooker recipes in Chapter 3, Paleo Spinach Quiche (Chapter 7: Paleo Egg Breakfasts) or Paleo Blueberry Pancakes (Chapter 8: Paleo Pancakes and Waffles).

There are also plenty of recipes that take just a moment to prepare and can be enjoyed on the run, such as the Paleo Strawberry-Banana Smoothie (Chapter 4: Paleo Shakes and Smoothies) or the nutrient-packed Paleo Granola Bars (Chapter 10: Paleo Breakfast Bars).

There's a recipe here for everyone, including the littlest cave people (Chapter 5: Paleo Breakfasts for Kids) and those who don't eat eggs (Chapter 9: Paleo Eggless Breakfasts).

In addition, in Chapter 2, you'll find some great tips for transitioning to the Paleo and gluten-free lifestyle, plus a great deal of information on why this transition could be the best decision you make for your health. Chapter 11 provides additional information about gluten and the science behind the Paleo diet. A helpful glossary of terms is included at the back of the book.

Enjoy the delicious breakfast recipes you'll find in these pages. More important, enjoy the health and well-being that the Paleo lifestyle provides.

WHY EAT A PALEO BREAKFAST?

A great deal of research has shown that eating a healthy breakfast is extremely important for weight management, maintaining a healthy blood sugar level, mental focus, and many other desirable benefits.

Unfortunately, because our lives are so busy and our schedules so unrelenting, many of us skip breakfast altogether or rely on a cup of coffee to start our day. Those of us who do eat breakfast often sit down to a bowl of cereal laden with sugar, high-fructose corn syrup, and very little nutrition. Others get their breakfast at the drive-thru—generally, highly processed foods full of unhealthy fats and plenty of sugar.

A healthy breakfast should include several key things:

- A good serving of high-quality protein to help you feel full, feed your muscles, and slow the absorption of carbohydrates for a steady supply of energy
- Healthy fats to help your body metabolize micronutrients, help you to feel full and satisfied, and support cognitive function throughout the morning
- Plenty of fiber to aid healthy digestion, provide energy, and help you to feel satisfied all morning long

No matter how busy you may be, you don't have to choose between an unhealthy breakfast and no breakfast at all.

The Paleo breakfast is a great way to start the day, even if you normally don't have time for a real meal. There are many ways to make time for a healthy Paleo breakfast. The recipes in this book offer lots of options for even the busiest families.

Many of the recipes take just a few minutes to prepare, a number of them can be made ahead of time, and quite a few can be enjoyed on the run. With so many healthful Paleo options, there's no need to start the day on an empty stomach or fill your body with drive-thru meals that offer little in the way of good nutrition.

What's on the Menu for Your Paleo Breakfast?

The Paleo diet is far from limiting and uninteresting. Although processed foods, grains, cereals, and sugar are out, there are still plenty of great foods to eat for breakfast. All vegetables are allowed on the diet except corn (it's a grain) and white potatoes (they're too starchy). All fruits are allowed and should be enjoyed as much as possible for their vitamin content, fiber, and natural sweetness.

Even though grains are off-limits, you can still enjoy delicious breakfast favorites, such as muffins, breakfast bars, pancakes, and waffles. These foods are made Paleo-friendly through the use of nut and seed flours, and they taste wonderful. They also pack a lot more nutrition than the traditional versions.

The focus on meats and eggs on the Paleo diet means you get plenty of protein and healthy fats in your morning meal, which is a very good thing. Protein and healthy fats help you to feel full so that you can avoid those mid-morning cravings for donuts and other junk food sitting around the office. They also slow the absorption of sugar into the bloodstream, which can help you to feel focused and energized without facing a sugar crash later on.

Try not to think that you're limited to "breakfast foods" for your morning meal. Many people on the Paleo diet have a breakfast that looks more like a traditional dinner: perhaps a serving of chicken and some vegetables. However, there are still plenty of more traditional breakfast options available to you on the Paleo diet.

You can prepare meals featuring all types of fruits and vegetables, most meats (including sausage), and items like muffins and pancakes made from nut and seed flours. Almond milk and coconut milk are excellent substitutions for cow's milk and can be used to drink, to prepare breakfast smoothies, and on homemade cereals and granolas.

See Chapter 11 for a comprehensive list of the foods you'll enjoy on the Paleo diet. Among them are plenty of delicious and healthful ingredients for whipping up a tasty Paleo breakfast.

2

10 TIPS FOR ENJOYING A HEALTHY PALEO BREAKFAST

Transitioning into eating a healthy Paleo breakfast every morning isn't very difficult, but we've compiled some tips to help you make it as simple and enjoyable as possible, no matter how hectic your schedule is.

1. **Assess your current breakfast and morning habits, and identify where you can make changes.**

    You can easily substitute Paleo-friendly pancakes and waffles for the wheat-based ones you eat now by using coconut, hazelnut, and other nut-based flours. If you're a cereal-eater, homemade Paleo granolas are delicious and easy to make in large batches. If mornings are extremely frenetic on weekdays, you can prepare Paleo muffins, breakfast bars, and frittatas on the weekends to eat during the week, or you can just whip up quick and yummy smoothies.

2. **Do some prep in the evening to make breakfast a faster affair.**

    Chop vegetables for omelets, stir up some pancake batter, or make extra servings of meats in the evening while you're preparing dinner and that will streamline breakfast preparation the next day.

3. **Don't focus on calorie counting.**

    The Paleo diet often results in weight loss, but not because of calorie restrictions. Since the diet is based on nutritious whole foods and excludes processed ingredients and sugar, most people end up eating fewer calories automatically. Also, calories alone are not the sole reason for excess weight. Junk foods, starches, and sugars promote fat storage by creating hormonal imbalances, particularly in insulin, leptin, ghrelin, and cortisol.

4. **Think of all Paleo-friendly foods as potential breakfast ingredients.**

    There's no law that says you can't enjoy chicken, broccoli, or watermelon for breakfast. Healthy foods are healthy at any time of the day.

5. **Make a deal with yourself and your family to skip the drive-thru.**

    Agree to stop visiting the drive-thru for breakfast (as well as lunch and dinner), and start putting away that money for something everyone will enjoy, like a mini-vacation, some sports equipment, or a gym membership.

6. **Get off-limits foods out of the house.**

    You may not be able to control the temptations you face out in the rest of the world, but you can control what's in your own home. Pull the processed and sugary items and grain products out of the pantry. Share them with friends or donate them to a food bank that desperately needs them.

7. **Cut yourself some slack.**

    Don't get discouraged or down on yourself if you slip up. The only failure is in letting that slipup derail you completely. Just decide to eat more healthfully at the next meal or the next day.

8. **Experiment with new recipes as often as possible.**

   Trying new foods is fun and keeps you from becoming bored or falling into a rut. This is an especially good idea if you have kids. If they don't like one pancake recipe, they may love the next one, and offering meals full of variety ensures balanced nutrition for the whole family.

9. **Pay attention to how you feel after eating a healthy Paleo breakfast.**

   It only takes a few days to notice how much more energized, focused, and satisfied you feel when you eat a healthy Paleo breakfast each morning. Focus on that sense of well-being when an unhealthy craving rears its head.

10. **Make your transition an adventure.**

    Try one or two new varieties of fruits, vegetables, or meats each week. If you have children, let each child choose one new ingredient or meal to try. This turns eating new food into a game and also introduces you (and your kids) to different flavors, textures, and colors.

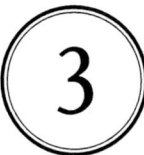

PALEO SLOW COOKER BREAKFASTS

Steamed Hazelnut Breakfast Bread

This recipe is a bit like a lighter version of steamed brown bread. The hazelnut flour, walnuts, and almond milk give it a deliciously nutty flavor with a hint of sweetness. It's perfect for breakfast or a snack.

- 1 to 1½ cups hot water
- 1½ cups hazelnut flour
- 1 teaspoon baking soda
- ½ teaspoon ground cinnamon
- ½ teaspoon ground nutmeg
- ½ teaspoon sea salt
- 1 cup plain almond milk
- ⅓ cup raw honey
- ½ cup chopped walnuts
- 1 teaspoon walnut oil

Turn the slow cooker on low heat and pour in enough hot water to reach a depth of about 1 inch. Place a cake or grilling rack in the slow cooker or use 4 fist-sized balls of aluminum foil as a homemade rack. Place the lid on the slow cooker.

In a large mixing bowl, combine the hazelnut flour, baking soda, cinnamon, nutmeg, and salt, and mix with a wooden spoon or whisk until well blended. Add the almond milk and honey, and mix just until combined. Do not overmix. Fold in the walnuts and stir until incorporated.

Grease a 2-quart soufflé dish or deep casserole with the walnut oil, and pour in the batter, spreading it evenly. Cover with foil and place the dish on the rack in the slow cooker.

Cover and cook on low heat for 3 hours, or until a toothpick inserted into the center of the bread comes out clean. Carefully remove both the dish and rack, remove the foil, and cool the dish on the rack for 10 to 15 minutes. Loosen the edges of the bread with a knife, transfer the bread to the rack, and let cool for 10 minutes before slicing. Wrap leftover bread in plastic wrap and store at room temperature for up to 3 days.

Serves 8.

Slow Cooker Almond Bread

This lightly scented almond bread is delicious, and it fits the Paleo-breakfast plan perfectly. Applesauce makes for a tender and moist bread, while toasted almonds add crunch and flavor. One bite and this is sure to become a favorite.

- Coconut oil or unsalted grass-fed butter for greasing
- 2 cups blanched almond flour
- 1 teaspoon baking soda
- 1 teaspoon sea salt
- ½ cup (1 stick) unsalted grass-fed butter, softened
- 1 cup raw honey
- 2 large eggs
- 1 cup unsweetened applesauce
- 3 tablespoons almond milk
- 1 tablespoon pure almond extract
- ½ cup sliced almonds, toasted

Lightly grease the slow cooker crock with coconut oil or butter.

In a large bowl, combine the almond flour, baking soda, and salt. Stir well and set aside.

In a separate bowl, using a mixer, beat the butter with the honey. Add the eggs, 1 at a time, beating after each addition. On low speed, beat in the applesauce, followed by the almond milk and extract. Add the flour mixture and beat until just combined.

Pour the batter into the prepared crock. Sprinkle the toasted almonds over the top. Cover and cook on high heat for 2 hours. Check doneness by inserting a toothpick. If it's not done, continue cooking on high until a toothpick comes out clean.

Allow the bread to cool, remove from the slow cooker, and slice. Wrap leftover bread in plastic wrap and store at room temperature for up to 3 days.

Serves 8 to 10.

Toasted Coconut Bread

If you like the taste of coconut, you'll love this lightly sweet bread with toasted coconut on top. This is a wonderful treat to enjoy with a cup of coffee in the morning, and it makes an excellent airy dessert as well. Be sure to use unsweetened shredded coconut for the topping, as sweetened varieties use refined sugar.

- Coconut oil or unsalted grass-fed butter for greasing
- 2 cups blanched almond flour
- 1 tablespoon coconut flour
- 1 teaspoon baking soda
- 1 teaspoon sea salt
- ½ cup coconut oil, melted
- 1 cup raw honey
- 2 large eggs
- 1 large ripe banana, mashed
- 3 tablespoons full-fat canned coconut milk
- 1 tablespoon pure vanilla extract
- ½ cup unsweetened shredded coconut, toasted

Lightly grease the slow cooker crock with coconut oil or butter.

In a large bowl, combine the almond flour, coconut flour, baking soda, and salt. Stir well and set aside.

In a separate bowl, using a mixer, beat the coconut oil with the honey. Add the eggs, 1 at a time, beating after each addition. On low speed, beat in the banana, followed by the coconut milk and vanilla. Add the flour mixture and beat until just combined.

Pour the batter into the prepared crock. Sprinkle the toasted coconut over the top. Cover and cook on high heat for 2 hours. Check doneness by inserting a toothpick. If it's not done, continue cooking on high until a toothpick comes out clean.

Allow the bread to cool, remove from the slow cooker, and slice. Wrap leftover bread in plastic wrap and store at room temperature for up to 3 days.

Serves 8 to 10.

Poached Pears with Cranberries

Sometimes you just want something sweet with your Paleo-friendly omelet. These poached pears fit the bill nicely, and they reheat well so you can make a large batch to have all week.

- 8 firm pears, such as Bosc, peeled and cored
- ½ teaspoon ground cinnamon
- ½ teaspoon ground nutmeg
- 2 tablespoons coconut oil
- ½ cup raw honey
- ½ teaspoon pure vanilla extract
- 1 cup dried, unsweetened cranberries

Cut a very thin slice from the bottom of each pear so the fruit will sit flat and steady.

In a small dish or bowl, combine the cinnamon and nutmeg, and sprinkle over the pears. Place the pears upright in the slow cooker.

Combine the coconut oil and honey in a small saucepan. Warm over low heat just until melted. Remove from the heat and stir in the vanilla. Pour the mixture over the pears and add the cranberries to the slow cooker, distributing them evenly around the pears.

Cover and cook on low heat for 4 hours. To serve, place a pear on a small plate, spoon cranberries around it, and drizzle a little of the cooking liquid on top.

Serves 8.

Dried Berry Compote

This easy compote makes a great topping for Paleo pancakes or waffles (see Chapter 8) on the weekends. It keeps well in the fridge for about 1 week in an airtight jar or dish.

- ½ cup raw honey
- ½ teaspoon pure vanilla extract
- ½ teaspoon pure almond extract
- ½ teaspoon ground cinnamon
- ½ teaspoon ground cloves
- 1 cup dried, unsweetened Bing cherries
- ½ cup dried, unsweetened blueberries
- ½ cup dried, unsweetened cranberries

In a medium saucepan over low heat, combine the honey, vanilla and almond extracts, cinnamon, and cloves. Cook, stirring frequently, until the honey is just melted.

Stir in the cherries, blueberries, and cranberries until well coated, and pour the mixture into the slow cooker. Cover and cook on low heat for 8 hours or overnight.

Serve warm over pancakes or waffles, or as a side dish.

Serves 6.

Cuban Pork and Plantain *Ropa Vieja*–Style Hash

Ropa vieja is a popular Cuban classic made of shredded beef or pork. In Cuban restaurants, it's most often served as a lunch or dinner entrée, but in homes, it also doubles as a filling breakfast with scrambled eggs.

- 1 teaspoon ground cumin
- 1 teaspoon garlic powder
- 1 teaspoon sea salt
- ½ teaspoon freshly ground black pepper
- 1 (1 ½-pound) pork sirloin roast, trimmed of visible fat
- 1 teaspoon olive oil
- ½ cup beef broth
- 1 bay leaf
- 4 plantains, peeled and cut in half

Combine the cumin, garlic powder, salt, and pepper in a small bowl, and rub all over the roast, coating it evenly.

In a large heavy skillet, heat the olive oil over medium-high heat. Brown the roast on all sides, 3 to 4 minutes per side. Set the skillet aside.

Place the roast in the slow cooker, and add the beef broth and bay leaf. Cover and cook on low heat for 8 hours.

Meanwhile, brown the plantains in the skillet over medium-high heat, using the leftover juices from the roast. Set aside.

After the pork has cooked for 4 hours, add the plantains to the slow cooker, arranging them around the roast. Continue cooking for 4 hours.

Transfer the roast to a cutting board to cool until it can be handled comfortably. While it cools, discard the bay leaf, dice the plantains, and set them aside in a large bowl.

Use clean hands or 2 forks to shred the pork, and combine with the plantains. To serve, ladle over or serve with scrambled eggs.

Serves 6.

Slow Cooker Pumpkin Butter

Pumpkin and apple butters add a bit of sweetness to the Paleo diet. They're extremely easy to make in the slow cooker and are delicious served warm after cooking overnight. Pumpkin butter, stored in an airtight jar, keeps well in the fridge for about 1 week.

- 2 (15-ounce) cans pumpkin puree (not pie filling)
- ½ cup unsweetened apple juice
- ½ cup raw honey
- ½ teaspoon ground allspice
- ½ teaspoon ground nutmeg
- ½ teaspoon ground ginger
- ½ teaspoon sea salt

In a medium bowl, combine the pumpkin puree, apple juice, and honey, and stir until well blended. Add the allspice, nutmeg, ginger, and salt, and stir well.

Pour the mixture into the slow cooker, cover, and cook on low heat for 8 hours. If the butter is a bit thin, uncover and increase the temperature to high heat. Allow the butter to reduce for about 30 minutes.

To serve, spread over Paleo-friendly breads, pancakes, or waffles, or use as a dip for fresh apple or pear slices.

Serves 12.

Vegetable Frittata

Frittatas become Paleo-friendly very easily. Though they're quick to make using the traditional cooking method, having one ready and waiting in the slow cooker for you when you wake up is especially nice.

- 12 large eggs, beaten
- ½ cup plain almond milk
- ½ cup diced red bell pepper
- ½ cup diced green bell pepper
- 1 medium white onion, diced
- 1 cup sliced white mushrooms
- 1 teaspoon sea salt
- ½ teaspoon freshly ground black pepper
- ½ teaspoon ground cumin
- 1 tablespoon olive oil

In a medium bowl, whisk the eggs and almond milk until well blended. Add the peppers, onion, and mushrooms. Mix well. Stir in the salt, pepper, and cumin.

Grease the bottom and halfway up the sides of the slow cooker crock with the olive oil. Pour in the egg mixture, cover, and cook on low heat for 8 hours. Serve warm with fresh fruit or Paleo-friendly muffins.

Serves 6.

Sweet Potato and Chicken-Sausage Hash

Commercially cured sausage is off-limits to most Paleo followers, but there are several organic sausage brands that are fresh rather than cured and therefore perfectly acceptable. This recipe uses chicken sausage, which is one of the easier types to find.

- 1 pound chicken sausage, casing removed
- 4 large sweet potatoes, peeled and grated
- 2 firm apples, peeled, cored, and chopped
- 1 small white onion, diced
- ¼ cup chicken broth or stock

In a large bowl, crumble the chicken sausage and combine with the sweet potatoes. Stir in the apples and onion, and press the mixture into the bottom of the slow cooker. Pour the broth over the top, cover, and cook on low heat for 8 hours or on high for 4 hours.

Serve the hash on its own or with eggs.

Serves 6.

PALEO SHAKES AND SMOOTHIES

Paleo Green Smoothie

Green drinks have become enormously popular, thanks to their dense concentration of many vital nutrients. Having a green smoothie for breakfast means you can get a great dose of nutrition no matter how hurried you may be.

- 1 cup cold water
- 1 cup diced cucumber
- 1 cup fresh baby spinach leaves
- 2 stalks celery, diced
- 1 large green apple, cored and diced
- 1 tablespoon lemon juice
- 1 teaspoon raw honey

Combine the water, cucumber, spinach, celery, and apple in a blender, and blend on high until smooth.

Add the lemon juice and honey, then blend on high for 30 seconds.

Pour into glasses and serve immediately.

Makes 2 large or 4 small smoothies.

Paleo Strawberry-Banana Smoothie

This smoothie is a breakfast favorite for kids and those who like something sweet to start the day, but it's also healthy and filling. You can freeze servings in individual airtight containers for about 2 hours and it becomes a frozen treat.

- 1 pint strawberries, stemmed
- 2 large bananas, sliced
- 1 teaspoon raw honey
- 1 teaspoon pure vanilla extract
- 3 cups coconut milk or plain almond milk
- Handful of ice cubes

Combine the strawberries, bananas, honey, and vanilla in a blender, and blend on high until smooth.

Turn the blender on low and gradually pour in the milk until it is fully incorporated.

Add the ice cubes, turn blender on high, and blend until thick and creamy. Serve immediately or freeze.

Makes 4 large or 8 small smoothies.

Protein Power Paleo Shake

This breakfast shake not only tastes great, but also delivers plenty of protein and heart-healthy fats. This is a rib-sticking shake that will power you through your busiest mornings.

- 2 cups plain almond milk
- ¼ cup almond butter
- 1 tablespoon raw honey
- 2 teaspoons ground flaxseed
- ½ teaspoon ground nutmeg
- 1 cup ripe avocado
- Handful of ice cubes

Combine the almond milk, almond butter, honey, flaxseed, and nutmeg in a blender, and blend on high until smooth.

Add the avocado and ice cubes and blend on high until thick and creamy. Serve immediately.

Makes 2 large or 4 small shakes.

Berrylicious Breakfast Smoothie

Frozen berries work just as well as fresh berries in this recipe. Be sure that they have not been sweetened with added sugar. This breakfast smoothie is a hit with kids and is loaded with antioxidants and vitamin C.

- 1½ cups berries (any combination of blueberries, blackberries, and raspberries)
- 2 cups plain almond milk
- 1 teaspoon pure vanilla extract
- 1 teaspoon raw honey
- Handful of ice cubes

Put the berries in a blender and blend on high until smooth.

Add the almond milk, vanilla, honey, and ice cubes, and blend on high until thick and creamy. Serve immediately.

Makes 2 large or 4 small smoothies.

Tropical Island Shake

When you want something that makes you feel like you're basking on a beautiful beach, this will do the trick. Similar to a piña colada, this shake is full of the flavors of summer.

- 1 cup cream of coconut
- 1 cup unsweetened canned pineapple
- ½ cup canned pineapple juice
- 1 teaspoon lime juice
- Handful of ice cubes

Combine the cream of coconut, pineapple and juice, and lime juice in a blender, and blend on high until smooth.

Add the ice cubes and blend on high until thick and creamy. Serve immediately.

Makes 2 large or 4 small shakes.

Nutty Carob Breakfast Smoothie

This smoothie is rich with the flavors of almond and carob. It's a great smoothie for breakfast but also makes a nice treat for those times when you crave a chocolate shake.

- 2 cups plain almond milk
- 2 tablespoons carob powder
- 2 tablespoons almond butter
- ½ teaspoon ground cinnamon
- Handful of ice cubes

Combine the almond milk, carob powder, almond butter, and cinnamon in a blender, and blend on high until smooth.

Add the ice cubes and blend on high until thick and creamy. Serve immediately.

Makes 2 large or 4 small smoothies.

Green Power Morning Smoothie

Kale is one of the most nutritious of the dark leafy greens, but it can be a little bitter in its raw form. The use of fresh orange juice and pears in this smoothie adds just the right touch of acidity and sweetness to satisfy.

- 1 cup fresh orange juice
- 1 cup chopped kale
- 1 cup chopped spinach
- 2 fresh pears, cored and chopped
- Handful of ice cubes

Combine the orange juice, kale, spinach, and pears in a blender, and blend on high until smooth.

Add the ice cubes and blend on high until thick and creamy. Serve immediately.

Makes 2 large or 4 small smoothies.

Bright Day Citrus Smoothie

The flavors of this sweet and tangy smoothie are similar to the classic orange sherbet-vanilla ice-cream treat, but this drink is far better for you. It will separate if it sits for too long, so be sure to drink it right away.

- 2 cups coconut milk or plain almond milk
- ¼ cup unsweetened frozen orange juice concentrate
- 1 banana, sliced
- 1 teaspoon pure vanilla extract
- Handful of ice cubes

Combine the milk, orange juice concentrate, banana, and vanilla in a blender, and blend on high until smooth.

Add the ice cubes and blend on high until thick and creamy. Serve immediately.

Makes 2 large or 4 small smoothies.

Key Lime Smoothie

If you like the taste of key lime pie, you'll love this smoothie. Loaded with vitamin C, a good amount of protein, and healthy fats, it's a wholesome drink that tastes like dessert.

- 2 cups coconut milk
- ¼ cup key lime juice
- ¼ cup raw honey
- 2 scoops egg white powder
- 1 teaspoon ground flaxseed

Combine all the ingredients in a blender and blend until smooth. Serve immediately.

Makes 2 large or 4 small smoothies.

PALEO BREAKFASTS FOR KIDS

Waffles with Strawberry Compote

The only thing kids love more than waffles is waffles topped with tons of warm strawberries in their own syrup. Make the compote in advance and double the batch. It's also wonderful served over Paleo-friendly ice cream or in a breakfast smoothie.

For the compote:
- 3 cups sliced fresh strawberries
- 2 tablespoons raw honey
- ½ teaspoon lemon juice
- Pinch of salt

For the waffles:
- 1 cup coconut flour
- ½ cup tapioca flour
- 1 teaspoon baking soda
- ¼ teaspoon salt
- 4 large eggs, beaten
- ⅓ cup plain coconut milk
- 2 tablespoons coconut oil, melted
- 1 teaspoon pure vanilla extract

To make the strawberry compote:
Combine the strawberries, honey, lemon juice, and salt in a small saucepan or skillet, and cook over low heat for 30 to 40 minutes, or until the strawberries are mostly broken down and a fairly thick syrup has formed. Keep warm until ready to use.

To make the waffles:

In a large mixing bowl, stir together the coconut and tapioca flours, baking soda, and salt until well blended.

In a separate bowl, mix together the eggs, coconut milk, coconut oil, and vanilla; then stir into the dry ingredients. Using a hand mixer, mix on low speed until well blended. Set aside for 10 minutes while heating the waffle iron.

Ladle batter into the waffle iron and cook according to manufacturer's instructions. As each waffle is finished, transfer it to a covered dish to keep warm.

To serve, top the warm waffles with the strawberry compote.

Makes 4 waffles.

Banana Nut Pops

A healthy breakfast doesn't necessarily have to be hot; in fact, this one is frozen. Make a bunch of these pops ahead of time and keep them in the freezer, not only for a quick breakfast but for an afterschool treat that kids love. They also love to help make these, so have the kids join you in the kitchen!

- 4 large just-ripe bananas
- 4 Popsicle sticks
- ½ cup almond butter
- 2 tablespoons raw honey
- ¾ cup chopped pecans

Peel and cut one end from each banana, and insert a Popsicle stick into the cut end.

In a small bowl, stir together the almond butter and honey, and heat in the microwave for 10 to 15 seconds, or just until the mixture is slightly thinned. Pour onto a sheet of wax paper or aluminum foil and spread with a spatula.

On another piece of wax paper or foil, spread the chopped pecans. Line a small baking sheet or large plate with a third piece of wax paper or foil.

Roll each banana first in the honey mixture until well coated, then in the nuts until completely covered, pressing down gently so the nuts adhere.

Place each finished banana onto the baking sheet. When all of the bananas have been coated, place the sheet in the freezer for at least 2 hours. For long-term storage, transfer the frozen bananas into a resealable plastic bag.

Makes 4 pops.

Yummy Paleo Granola

If your kids are like most other kids, they equate breakfast with a crunchy bowl of cold cereal. This homemade and Paleo-friendly granola has all the crunch and sweetness kids look for in their cereal bowl, but is much better for them than the commercial product. The granola will keep in an airtight container for up to a month.

- 1 cup chopped walnuts
- 1 cup raw pumpkin seeds (or roasted)
- 1 cup unsweetened coconut flakes
- ½ teaspoon salt
- ½ teaspoon ground cinnamon
- ½ teaspoon ground nutmeg
- ½ cup coconut oil, melted
- ½ cup raw honey, melted
- 1 teaspoon pure vanilla extract
- 1 cup dried cranberries
- 1 cup dried apricots, roughly chopped

Preheat the oven to 325 degrees F. Line a baking sheet with aluminum foil.

In a large bowl, combine the walnuts, pumpkin seeds, and coconut flakes, and mix until well blended. Add the salt, cinnamon, and nutmeg and mix well.

In a small measuring cup, combine the melted coconut oil and honey and vanilla, then pour over the nut mixture. Add the cranberries and apricots.

Lightly grease your hands with coconut oil, and mix the granola until all the ingredients are well coated.

Spread the granola in a thin layer on the baking sheet. Bake for 30 minutes, or until the nuts and coconut are golden, stirring once after 15 minutes.

Allow the granola to cool for about 5 minutes, until still warm but cool enough to handle. Crumble the granola, and let it to cool to room temperature. Store in an airtight container.

Serves 12.

Egg and Sausage Muffins

Kids seem to love anything that's baked in a muffin pan, and these hearty egg and sausage cups are no exception. They will keep in the fridge for up to 2 days but don't freeze well.

- ½ pound nitrate-free sausage (or about 10 sausage patties, chopped)
- 10 large eggs, beaten
- 2 tablespoons plain almond or coconut milk
- ¾ cup Paleo-friendly bread crumbs
- 1 teaspoon dried parsley

Preheat the oven to 350 degrees F.

In a heavy skillet, brown the sausage over medium-high heat, stirring frequently to break it up, for about 10 minutes, or until cooked through.

Drain the sausage, reserving about 1 tablespoon of the drippings for the pan, and use a pastry brush to grease the bottoms and edges of an 8-cup muffin pan.

In a medium mixing bowl, combine the eggs and almond milk, then stir in the sausage.

In a small bowl, combine the bread crumbs and parsley.

Divide the egg mixture between the muffin cups, filling them about two-thirds full.

Top each muffin cup with some of the bread crumb mixture, and bake for 30 to 35 minutes, until the eggs are completely set.

Allow the egg muffins to cool for about 5 minutes, then run a knife around the edges and remove from the pan. To serve, place two egg muffins on each plate and serve warm.

Makes 8 egg muffins.

Coconut-Pineapple Pancakes

These pancakes are delightfully different, with fresh pineapple giving them a yummy bit of tropical flavor that kids love.

- 1 pineapple, cored
- 1 cup coconut flour
- 2 teaspoons baking soda
- ½ teaspoon salt
- 2 cups plain coconut milk
- 8 large eggs, beaten
- 4 teaspoons raw honey, divided
- 1 teaspoon pure vanilla extract
- 1 tablespoon coconut oil, divided

Cut the pineapple in half horizontally. Cut one of the halves into slices and set aside. Roughly chop the other half. Place the chopped pineapple on a plate lined with paper towels, cover with another paper towel, and squeeze out any excess juice.

In a large mixing bowl, stir together the coconut flour, baking soda, and salt.

In a separate bowl, whisk together the coconut milk, eggs, 2 teaspoons of the honey, and the vanilla until well blended. Stir in the chopped pineapple. Fold the mixture into the dry ingredients and stir just until a lumpy batter forms. Set aside for 10 minutes.

In a medium heavy skillet, melt a dime-size portion of the coconut oil over medium heat.

Ladle enough pancake batter into the skillet to make a 3- to 4-inch pancake. Cook the pancakes one or two at a time for 3 minutes on the first side, or until bubbles form at the edges, then flip over and cook for 1 minute. As the pancakes are cooked, stack them on a plate and cover to keep warm.

Cook the remaining batter, adding more coconut oil to the skillet as needed.

Meanwhile, preheat the broiler and line a baking sheet with aluminum foil.

Brush the pineapple slices with the remaining 2 teaspoons honey, and broil for 3 to 4 minutes, or just until golden.

To serve, stack a few pancakes on each plate and top with pineapple slices.

Serves 4.

Chocolate-Banana Breakfast Shake

Kids enjoy shakes and smoothies anytime of the day, and one of their favorite combinations is chocolate and banana. This breakfast shake packs lots of nutrition, but all they'll notice is the creamy goodness.

- 3 ripe medium bananas, broken into pieces
- 2 cups plain almond milk
- 2 tablespoons almond butter
- 1 tablespoon cocoa powder
- 1 teaspoon raw honey
- 1 teaspoon pure vanilla extract
- Handful of ice cubes

In a blender, combine the bananas, almond milk, almond butter, cocoa powder, honey, and vanilla, and blend on high until smooth.

Add the ice cubes and blend until thick and creamy.

Serves 4.

Paleo Eggs Benedict

Eggs Benedict is a classic recipe that is also a pretty unhealthy one. This recipe uses Paleo hollandaise sauce and Paleo-friendly toast to make it a delicious alternative to the fat- and grain-heavy original. Kids can't get enough!

For the eggs Benedict:
- 1 quart water with 1 tablespoon vinegar
- 4 large eggs
- 1 cup frozen chopped spinach, thawed and well drained, or fresh spinach
- 4 thin slices nitrate-free ham
- 4 slices toasted Paleo-friendly bread or 4 medium Paleo-friendly savory muffins

For the hollandaise sauce:
- 4 large egg yolks
- ¼ cup light olive oil
- 3 tablespoons hot water
- 1 teaspoon lemon juice
- ¼ teaspoon dry mustard
- ¼ teaspoon salt
- ¼ teaspoon freshly ground black pepper

To make the eggs Benedict:

Bring the water and vinegar to a boil. Carefully break in one egg at a time, swirling each egg around the pan a few times gently with a rubber spoon or spatula. Reduce the heat to low and cover the pan. Continue cooking the eggs for about 4 minutes, or until the yolks are almost cooked through. Use a slotted spoon to transfer the eggs to a shallow bowl. Cover to keep warm.

Meanwhile, heat the spinach and ham slices in the microwave for about 2 minutes, or until heated through. Cover to keep warm.

To make the hollandaise sauce:

In a double boiler or a metal mixing bowl set over boiling water (but not touching it), whisk together the eggs yolks and olive oil. Slowly whisk in the hot water, then add the lemon juice, dry mustard, salt, and pepper, whisking continuously for 1 minute, until it has thickened.

Place a slice of toast on each plate, and top with a quarter of the spinach and one slice of ham. Top with one poached egg and pour a quarter of the sauce on top.

Serves 4.

Eggs on Sweet Potato Rounds

Kids love the taste of sweet potatoes and that's a great thing—they're loaded with protein, fiber, and beta-carotene. Not only is this fun to eat, it's good for them, too. Bake the sweet potatoes the night before while you're cooking dinner.

- 2 tablespoons chopped pancetta or unsmoked bacon
- 2 large baked sweet potatoes
- ½ teaspoon salt
- ¼ teaspoon freshly ground black pepper
- 4 large eggs

In a large heavy skillet, brown the pancetta over medium heat for 6 to 8 minutes, or until cooked thoroughly. Use a slotted spoon to transfer the pancetta to a paper towel and drain the skillet of all but 1 teaspoon of drippings.

Meanwhile, use a spoon to scoop the flesh from the sweet potatoes and place it in a medium mixing bowl. Use a fork to mix in the salt and pepper.

Heat the skillet over medium-high heat until the drippings are sizzling. Scoop 4 mounds of mashed sweet potato into the skillet, using about ¼ cup of mashed sweet potato for each.

Use the back of an ice-cream scoop to form a deep well in the center of each sweet potato round, deep enough so the pan is visible. Crack an egg into the center of each round, cover the pan, and cook for 4 to 5 minutes, or until the egg whites are completely set but the yolks are still somewhat runny. Sprinkle with cooked pancetta or bacon.

Transfer one potato round to each plate with a spatula and serve.

Serves 4.

6

PALEO BREAKFAST MUFFINS

Paleo Blueberry Muffins

Think you have to give up your morning blueberry muffin just because you've gone Paleo? Think again. These moist muffins, bursting with juicy blueberries, will satisfy your craving for a coffee shop muffin without the guilt that usually accompanies it. Freeze them for a quick breakfast or sweet treat anytime you want.

- 2½ cups blanched almond flour
- 1 tablespoon coconut flour
- 1 teaspoon baking soda
- 1 teaspoon sea salt
- 1 teaspoon ground cinnamon
- 1 stick unsalted grass-fed butter, softened
- 1 cup pure maple syrup
- 2 large eggs
- 2 cups unsweetened applesauce, preferably homemade
- ¼ cup unsweetened almond milk
- 1 tablespoon pure vanilla extract
- 1 cup fresh or frozen blueberries

Preheat the oven to 350 degrees F.

In a large bowl, add the almond flour, coconut flour, baking soda, salt, and cinnamon, and stir well to combine.

In a mixing bowl, beat the butter with the maple syrup until smooth. Add the eggs one at a time, beating to incorporate after each addition. On low speed, add the applesauce, almond milk, and vanilla.

Add the dry ingredients to the liquid mixture, and beat on low speed until just combined. Carefully fold in the blueberries. Stir gently until well combined.

Line two 6-cup muffin pans with liners, and fill each cup two-thirds full. Bake for 12 to 14 minutes, or until the muffin tops are golden brown. Cool on a rack, then loosen the muffins with a knife, and serve.

Store muffins in an airtight container for up to 3 days.

Makes 1 dozen muffins.

Paleo "Bran" Muffins

While these muffins don't actually contain bran (the outer bran of the wheat stalk is not gluten-free or Paleo-friendly), flaxseed and molasses give them the same color, texture, and flavor of your favorite coffee shop bran muffin. They contain no wheat or refined carbs, so you're getting something delicious without the wheat belly that comes from eating the traditional bran muffins. Try them plain or with Paleo-approved jam for an easy and healthful breakfast.

- ½ cup blanched almond flour
- ½ cup ground flaxseed
- 2 tablespoons coconut flour
- 1 teaspoon baking soda
- ½ teaspoon sea salt
- 1 tablespoon natural almond butter
- 3 large eggs
- 2 tablespoons molasses
- 1 small ripe banana, mashed
- ½ cup unsweetened almond milk

Preheat the oven to 350 degrees F.

In a large bowl, combine the almond flour, flaxseed, coconut flour, baking soda, and salt.

In a separate bowl, beat together the almond butter, eggs, molasses, mashed banana, and almond milk. Pour the wet ingredients into the flour mixture, and stir until well combined.

Line two 6-cup muffin pans with liners, and fill each cup two-thirds full. Bake for 12 to 14 minutes, or until the muffin tops are golden brown. Cool on a rack, then loosen the muffins with a knife, and serve.

Store muffins in an airtight container for up to 3 days.

Makes 1 dozen muffins.

"Oatmeal" Muffins

You've probably been told that a bowl of hot oatmeal is one of the best ways to start your day. However, if you've gone Paleo, oats aren't on the menu. Don't worry, these muffins will satisfy the craving. Finely shredded coconut mimics the texture of oats, and the cinnamon and maple syrup will remind you of that winter bowl of oatmeal. These muffins are good at room temperature, but they're at their best when served warm.

- 2 cups blanched almond flour
- ½ cup unsweetened shredded coconut
- ½ teaspoon sea salt
- 1 teaspoon ground cinnamon
- 2 teaspoons baking soda
- 3 large eggs
- ½ cup coconut oil, melted
- ¼ cup pure maple syrup
- ½ cup unsweetened almond milk

Preheat the oven to 350 degrees F.

In a large bowl, combine the almond flour, coconut, salt, cinnamon, and baking soda.

In a mixing bowl, beat the eggs with the coconut oil, maple syrup, and almond milk until light and smooth. Pour into the flour mixture, and stir until well combined.

Line two 6-cup muffin pans with liners, and fill each cup two-thirds full. Bake for 12 to 14 minutes, or until the muffin tops are a deep golden brown. Cool on a rack, then loosen the muffins with a knife, and serve.

Store muffins in an airtight container for up to 3 days. They will also keep for several weeks in the freezer in a resealabe airtight bag.

Makes 1 dozen muffins.

Apple Cranberry Breakfast Muffins

Looking for something sweet and tart to start your morning with? Look no further than these delightful breakfast muffins made with fresh cranberries and apples, and bursting with fresh fruit flavor. Combining chopped fresh cranberries with a bit of coconut sugar helps to offset their natural tartness.

- ½ cup fresh cranberries
- 2 tablespoons coconut sugar
- 2 tablespoons pure maple syrup
- 1 large egg
- 2 teaspoons pure vanilla extract
- 1 cup unsweetened almond milk
- 1 cup blanched almond flour
- ¼ teaspoon sea salt
- ¼ teaspoon baking soda
- 1 apple, peeled, cored, and chopped

Preheat the oven to 350 degrees F.

Put the cranberries in a food processor with the coconut sugar. Pulse until the cranberries are chopped and well combined with the sugar, but do not puree them.

In a mixing bowl, add the maple syrup, egg, vanilla, and almond milk, and beat to combine.

In a separate bowl, combine the almond flour, salt, and baking soda. Stir well. Add the wet ingredients and stir until well combined. Fold in the chopped cranberries and apples.

Line two 6-cup muffin pans with liners, and fill each cup two-thirds full. Bake for 12 to 14 minutes, or until the muffin tops are golden brown. Cool on a rack, then loosen the muffins with a knife, and serve warm or at room temperature.

Store muffins in an airtight container for up to 3 days.

Makes 1 dozen muffins.

Bacon and Roasted Pepper Muffins

These savory muffins are full of flavor from crispy bacon and roasted peppers, with a texture that is light and airy. They're great when you want something that's simple but isn't necessarily sweet. They also freeze well.

- 1 cup blanched almond flour
- ½ teaspoon sea salt
- 2 teaspoons baking soda
- 6 large eggs
- ½ cup unsalted grass-fed butter, melted and cooled
- ½ cup water
- 4 or 5 slices nitrate-free bacon, cooked until crisp and crumbled
- 1 roasted red pepper, finely chopped

Preheat the oven to 325 degrees F.

In a large bowl, combine the almond flour, salt, and baking soda.

In a mixing bowl, beat the eggs with the butter and water. Add in the bacon and pepper, and stir to combine. Pour the wet ingredients into the flour mixture, and stir until well combined.

Line two 6-cup muffin pans with liners, and fill each cup two-thirds full. Bake for 12 to 14 minutes, or until the muffin tops are golden brown. Cool on a rack, then loosen the muffins with a knife, and serve.

Store muffins in an airtight container for up to 3 days. They will also keep for several weeks in the freezer in a resealable airtight bag.

Makes 1 dozen muffins.

French Toast Muffins

These French toast muffins require Paleo-friendly bread and the result is well worth the effort. If you have a Paleo bread recipe, you can make your own. Set aside a few slices to use for these muffins—they are divine. Their flavor is best when served right from the oven.

For the topping:
- 1 large egg
- 3 tablespoons unsweetened almond milk
- 1 teaspoon pure vanilla extract
- ½ teaspoon ground cinnamon
- 4 slices Paleo-friendly white bread, cut into small cubes

For the muffins:
- 2 cups blanched almond flour
- ½ teaspoon sea salt
- 2 teaspoons baking soda
- 4 large eggs
- ½ cup unsalted grass-fed butter, melted and cooled
- ¼ cup raw honey
- ½ cup unsweetened almond milk
- Pure maple syrup, for brushing the muffins

To make the topping:
Beat the egg with the almond milk, vanilla, and cinnamon, and pour over the bread cubes. Set aside.

To make the muffins:
Preheat the oven to 350 degrees F.

In a large bowl, combine the almond flour, salt, and baking soda. Set aside.

In a mixing bowl, beat the eggs with the butter, honey, and almond milk until the mixture is light and smooth. Pour the wet ingredients into the flour mixture, and stir until well combined.

Line two 6-cup muffin pans with liners, and fill each cup two-thirds full. Sprinkle on the bread cube topping evenly between the cups. Bake for 12 to 14 minutes, or until the muffin tops are golden brown and the bread cubes are browned around the edges. Brush the tops with maple syrup and serve warm.

Makes 1 dozen muffins.

Paleo Morning Glory Muffins

These dense and delicious muffins are chock-full of goodness, perfect to start the day with or for a midday snack. Loaded with ingredients like carrots, raisins, and apples, this is not a cakelike muffin, but sweet and full of flavor and texture.

- 2 tablespoons coconut oil, melted
- ½ cup unsweetened almond milk
- 1 large egg
- 1 teaspoon pure vanilla extract
- 1 cup almond flour
- ¼ cup ground flaxseed
- ¼ cup unsweetened shredded coconut
- 1 tablespoon ground cinnamon
- ¼ teaspoon ground nutmeg
- 1 teaspoon baking soda
- 1 cup grated carrots
- 1 apple, peeled, cored, and chopped
- ¼ cup raisins
- ½ cup walnuts, chopped

Preheat the oven to 350 degrees F.

In a medium bowl, add the coconut oil, almond milk, egg, and vanilla, and stir well to combine.

In a separate bowl, whisk together the almond flour, flaxseed, coconut, cinnamon, nutmeg, and baking soda. Pour the wet ingredients into the flour mixture, and stir until just combined. Fold in the carrots, apple, raisins, and walnuts.

Line two 6-cup muffin pans with liners, and fill each cup two-thirds full. Bake for 12 to 14 minutes, or until the muffin tops are dark brown. Cool on a rack, then loosen the muffins with a knife, and serve.

Store muffins in an airtight container for up to 3 days.

Makes 1 dozen muffins.

Chai Spiced Muffins

Fragrant with a hint of Indian spices, these delicious muffins are an excellent substitute for your usual chai latte. They are a perfect quick breakfast or a sweet snack. Serve them warm with a pat of unsalted grass-fed butter.

- 2 cups blanched almond flour
- 2 teaspoons baking soda
- 1 teaspoon ground cinnamon
- ½ teaspoon ground ginger
- ½ teaspoon ground cardamom
- ¼ teaspoon freshly ground black pepper
- ½ teaspoon sea salt
- 4 large eggs
- ½ cup coconut oil, melted
- ¼ cup raw honey
- ½ cup unsweetened almond milk

Preheat the oven to 350 degrees F.

In a large bowl, combine the almond flour, baking soda, cinnamon, ginger, cardamom, pepper, and salt.

In a mixing bowl, beat the eggs with the coconut oil, honey, and almond milk until the mixture is light and smooth. Pour the wet ingredients into the flour mixture, and stir until well combined.

Line two 6-cup muffin pans with liners, and fill each cup two-thirds full. Bake for 12 to 14 minutes, or until muffin tops are golden brown. Cool on a rack, then loosen the muffins with a knife, and serve.

Store muffins in an airtight container for up to 3 days. They will also keep for several weeks in the freezer in a resealable airtight bag.

Makes 1 dozen muffins.

7

PALEO EGG BREAKFASTS

Paleo Spinach Quiche

Traditional quiche is usually loaded with cheese, but you won't miss it in this flavorful recipe. It's a great dish to make the night before, especially if you already have the oven on for dinner.

- 1 teaspoon olive oil, plus more for greasing the pan
- 1 cup chopped fresh spinach
- ½ cup chopped red onion
- ½ teaspoon salt
- ½ teaspoon freshly ground black pepper
- ½ teaspoon ground nutmeg
- 8 large eggs, beaten
- ½ cup plain almond milk

Preheat the oven to 350 degrees F. Grease a 9-inch glass pie plate.

In a small skillet, heat the olive oil over medium heat, and sauté the spinach, onion, salt, pepper, and nutmeg for about 5 minutes, or just until the onions are translucent.

Stir the eggs and almond milk together in a small bowl. Add the spinach mixture, stir, and pour the mixture into the pie plate.

Bake the quiche on the middle oven rack for 30 to 40 minutes, or until the center is completely set. Serve warm or at room temperature.

Serves 4 to 6.

Paleo Frittata

A frittata is a wonderfully versatile dish for the Paleo diet. Frittatas can be prepared using whatever vegetables or meats you have on hand for a quick one-skillet meal. They can also be made ahead and even frozen.

- 1 teaspoon olive oil
- 2 cloves garlic, chopped
- ½ cup chopped yellow onion
- ½ cup diced red bell pepper
- ½ cup sliced fresh mushrooms
- ½ cup chopped fresh spinach
- ½ teaspoon salt
- ¼ teaspoon freshly ground black pepper
- ½ teaspoon paprika
- 8 large eggs, beaten

In a large heavy skillet with a lid, heat the olive oil over medium heat, and sauté the garlic, onion, bell pepper, and mushrooms for about 5 minutes.

Add the spinach and season with salt, pepper, and paprika. Sauté for another 2 to 3 minutes, or until the bell peppers are fork-tender.

Reduce the heat to medium-low and pour the eggs over the vegetables. Cover the pan and cook for 7 to 9 minutes, or until the eggs are completely set and dry in the center.

Cut the frittata into wedges and serve with fresh fruit or a Paleo-friendly muffin.

Serves 4 to 6.

Italian Scramble

This recipe is great for the summertime, when vegetables are at their peak of flavor and freshness. Be sure to use fresh herbs. Even better, use herbs you've grown in your own window box.

- 1 teaspoon olive oil
- 2 cloves garlic, chopped
- ¼ cup diced red onion
- ¼ cup chopped fresh basil, plus more for garnish (optional)
- 2 tablespoons chopped fresh oregano
- ½ cup diced ripe tomato
- ½ teaspoon salt
- ¼ teaspoon freshly ground black pepper
- 8 large eggs, beaten

In a large heavy skillet, heat the olive oil over medium heat, and sauté the garlic, onion, basil, and oregano for 2 minutes, stirring occasionally.

Stir in the tomato, salt, and pepper until well combined, then pour in the eggs. Cook, stirring frequently, until the eggs are set, 3 to 4 minutes.

To serve, spoon onto plates and garnish with a little fresh basil, if desired.

Serves 4.

Paleo Western Omelet

Most Paleo diet guidelines exclude ham, bacon, and deli meats because of the nitrates and sugars that are usually added. However, you can eat unsmoked bacon, which is called pancetta and is easily found at the grocery store. It is more expensive, but a little bit goes a long way.

- ½ cup diced pancetta or unsmoked bacon
- 1 teaspoon olive oil (optional)
- ¼ cup diced green pepper
- ¼ cup diced red bell pepper
- ¼ cup diced white onion
- ¼ teaspoon salt (optional, depending on the saltiness of the pancetta)
- ¼ teaspoon freshly ground black pepper
- 6 large eggs, beaten

Place a medium heavy skillet over medium heat. Add the pancetta and cook, stirring occasionally, until it's nicely browned, 6 to 7 minutes.

If the pancetta is very lean and the skillet has little grease, add the olive oil. Then add the green and red bell peppers, onion, salt (if desired), and pepper. Sauté for 3 to 4 minutes, or until the bell peppers are almost fork-tender. Transfer the vegetables to a plate and set aside, leaving the oil in the pan.

Increase the heat to medium-high and pour in the eggs. Tilt the pan in a circular motion to spread them evenly around the pan. As the eggs cook, use a rubber spatula to pull the edges in toward the center, allowing runny egg to flow to the pan edge.

Cook until the center of the omelet is almost completely dry, 3 to 4 minutes, then use a spatula to flip the omelet over. Spoon the filling over one half of the omelet, and fold the other half over the filling. Immediately slide the omelet onto a cutting board.

To serve, slice the omelet in half and place each on a plate.

Serves 2.

Paleo Egg White Omelet

Omelets made with egg whites are just as nutritious and filling as those made with whole eggs. If you prefer not to eat egg yolks, this recipe is for you. Refrigerate the yolks if you separate whole eggs for this dish, and use them later in baking or to make Paleo mayonnaise (see the Paleo mayo recipe later in this chapter).

- 1 teaspoon olive oil
- 8 egg whites, lightly beaten
- ¼ teaspoon salt
- ¼ teaspoon freshly ground black pepper
- ¼ cup diced white onion
- ¼ cup diced tomato
- 2 tablespoons chopped fresh parsley
- Parsley sprigs, for garnish

In a medium heavy skillet, heat the olive oil over medium heat. Pour in the egg whites and tilt the skillet to spread them evenly around the pan. When the edges and center of the omelet are nearly dry, use a spatula to flip it over.

Season the omelet with the salt and pepper, then spread the onion, tomato, and chopped parsley over one half of the omelet. Cook for 1 minute, then fold the other half over the filling. Immediately slide the omelet onto a cutting board.

To serve, slice the omelet in half and place each on a plate. Garnish with parsley sprigs.

Serves 2.

Mushroom-Rosemary Omelet

Mushrooms and rosemary work beautifully together in this omelet. To save time, cook up a large batch of mushroom filling on the weekend or in the evening and keep it refrigerated for up to 1 week.

- 2 teaspoons olive oil, divided
- 1 pound sliced fresh mushrooms
- 2 cloves garlic
- ¼ cup sliced green onions
- 1 tablespoon chopped fresh rosemary
- ¼ teaspoon salt
- ¼ teaspoon freshly ground black pepper
- 6 large eggs, beaten
- Rosemary sprigs, for garnish

Heat 1 teaspoon of the olive oil in a medium heavy skillet over medium-high heat. Add the mushrooms and garlic, and cook, stirring frequently, for 5 minutes. Add the green onions, rosemary, salt, and pepper, and cook for 2 minutes. Transfer to a bowl and set aside.

Add the remaining 1 teaspoon of olive oil to the skillet and reduce the heat to medium. Pour in the eggs and tilt the skillet in a circular motion to spread them evenly around the pan. Cook for 3 to 5 minutes, using a spatula to pull the edges in toward the center and allowing runny egg to flow to the pan edge.

Once the center of the omelet is nearly dry, use a spatula to flip the omelet over. Spread the mushroom filling over one half of the omelet, and fold the other half over the filling. Immediately slide the omelet onto a cutting board.

To serve, cut the omelet in half and place each on a plate. Garnish with rosemary sprigs.

Serves 2.

Paleo Vegetable Omelet

This omelet is loaded with colorful fresh vegetables. Feel free to mix and add whatever is on hand or at the peak of its season. To save time in the mornings, make the veggie filling the evening before or over the weekend, and refrigerate until needed. This makes four two-egg omelets—the perfect size for younger family members and lighter eaters.

- 3 teaspoons olive oil, divided
- ½ cup diced red bell pepper
- ½ cup diced yellow onion
- 1 small yellow squash, diced
- ½ cup sliced fresh mushrooms
- 1 cup fresh baby spinach leaves
- 2 tablespoons chopped fresh basil
- 2 tablespoons chopped fresh parsley
- ½ teaspoon salt
- ¼ teaspoon freshly ground black pepper
- 8 large eggs, beaten

In a medium heavy skillet, heat 1 teaspoon of the olive oil over medium-high heat. Add the bell pepper, onion, squash, and mushrooms, and cook, stirring frequently, for 3 to 4 minutes, or until the onions are translucent. Add the spinach, basil, parsley, salt, and pepper, and cook for 2 minutes, or just until the spinach is wilted.

Transfer the cooked vegetables to a plate lined with paper towels, and pour out any excess liquid in the pan.

Add 1 teaspoon of the olive oil to the skillet and heat. When hot, pour in half of the eggs. Tilt the skillet in a circular motion to spread them evenly over the pan. Cook for 3 to 5 minutes, using a spatula to pull the edges in toward the center and allowing runny egg to flow to the pan edge.

Once the center of the omelet is nearly dry, use a spatula to flip the omelet over. Spread half of the vegetable filling over one half of the omelet, and fold the other half over the filling.

Immediately slide onto a cutting board. Repeat to make the second omelet with the remaining olive oil, eggs, and filling.

To serve, cut each omelet in half and place each on a plate.

Serves 4.

Paleo Spinach Omelet

Spinach is loaded with iron and vitamins and it cooks very quickly. This omelet takes just a few minutes to prepare. Its simple flavors are delicious.

- 2 teaspoons olive oil, divided
- 1 cup fresh baby spinach leaves
- ¼ cup chopped white onion
- 2 cloves garlic, crushed
- ½ teaspoon salt
- ¼ teaspoon freshly ground black pepper
- 6 large eggs, beaten
- Parsley sprigs, for garnish

In a medium heavy skillet, heat 1 teaspoon of the olive oil over medium-high heat. Cook the spinach, onion, garlic, salt, and pepper for 3 to 4 minutes, or until the spinach is just wilted and onions are slightly translucent. Transfer the vegetables to a plate and set aside.

Add the remaining 1 teaspoon of olive oil to the skillet and heat. When hot, pour in the eggs. Tilt the skillet in a circular motion to spread them evenly around the pan. Cook for 3 to 5 minutes, using a spatula to pull the edges in toward the center and allowing runny egg to flow to the pan edge.

Once the center of the omelet is nearly dry, use a spatula to flip the omelet over. Spread the vegetable filling over one half of the omelet, then fold the other half over the filling. Immediately slide the omelet onto a cutting board.

To serve, cut the omelet in half and place each on a plate. Garnish with parsley sprigs.

Serves 2.

Paleo-Friendly Breakfast Egg Salad

This delicious and filling egg salad can also make a nice lunch sandwich, so be sure to make extra. Paleo mayo, once you use it in the egg salad, will keep for about 1 week.

For the Paleo mayo:
- 1 large egg, at room temperature
- 2 tablespoons lemon juice, at room temperature
- ¼ teaspoon salt
- ¼ teaspoon freshly ground black pepper
- 1¼ cups light olive oil, divided

For the egg salad:
- 8 hard-boiled egg yolks, mashed
- ½ teaspoon Dijon mustard
- 8 hard-boiled egg whites, diced
- ½ cup cooked and crumbled unsmoked bacon or pancetta
- 8 slices Paleo-friendly bread, toasted
- 4 romaine lettuce leaves
- 8 slices fresh tomato

To make the Paleo mayo:

Have both the egg and lemon juice at room temperature. This is very important for the recipe's success.

Put the egg, lemon juice, salt, pepper, and ¼ cup of the olive oil in a blender, and blend on medium speed until smooth.

Reduce to low speed, and very slowly drizzle the remaining 1 cup olive oil through the blender lid. This may take as long as 2 to 3 minutes.

Once the mayo is smooth and opaque, transfer to an airtight jar and refrigerate.

To make the egg salad:

Combine the egg yolks, 2 tablespoons of the Paleo mayo, and the Dijon mustard in a mixing bowl, and stir with a fork until well blended. Fold in the eggs whites and bacon, and stir just until incorporated.

Take four pieces of toast and put on each a lettuce leaf, two slices of tomato, and a quarter of the egg salad. Top each with another piece of toast to finish the sandwich.

To serve, cut each sandwich in half and serve with fresh fruit.

Makes 4 sandwiches.

Paleo Sausage Casserole

This casserole is both tasty and extremely convenient. You can put it together in the evening to pop into the oven the next morning, or you can cook the casserole ahead of time and reheat it. It's equally good served hot or at room temperature.

- 1 teaspoon olive oil
- 1 pound nitrate-free pork sausage
- 2 cups plain almond milk
- 12 large eggs
- 2 teaspoons dry mustard
- 1 teaspoon salt
- ½ teaspoon freshly ground black pepper
- 4 cups cubed day-old Paleo-friendly bread
- 2 tablespoons chopped fresh parsley

Grease a 9 x 13 inch glass baking dish with the olive oil and set aside.

In a large heavy skillet, cook the sausage over medium-high heat until browned, 7 to 9 minutes. Use a spatula to chop up and crumble the sausage while cooking.

With a slotted spoon, transfer the sausage to a plate lined with paper towels to drain, and let the sausage cool to room temperature.

Meanwhile, in a mixing bowl, combine the almond milk, eggs, dry mustard, salt, and pepper, and stir well.

Add the sausage and bread cubes to the egg mixture and blend well. Pour into the baking dish, top with the parsley, and cover with foil or plastic wrap. Refrigerate overnight.

Preheat the oven to 350 degrees F and position a rack in the center of the oven.

Bake the casserole, uncovered, for 50 to 60 minutes, or until a toothpick inserted into the center comes out clean.

To serve, cut the casserole into squares and serve with fresh fruit.

Serves 6.

8

PALEO PANCAKES AND WAFFLES

<u>Special note for pancake and waffle recipes:</u> It's important to have your eggs, liquids, and flours at room temperature before you begin preparing the pancake and waffle batters. This ensures that the batter is the right consistency for the lightest finished product.

Paleo Blueberry Pancakes

Pancakes made with nut flours are a delicious treat with a delicate flavor. They don't always hold together as well as wheat-based cakes, so make into 3- to 4-inch rounds for easier flipping.

- 2 cups hazelnut flour
- 2 cups fresh blueberries
- 4 large eggs, beaten
- ½ cup plain almond milk
- 1 teaspoon baking soda
- 1 teaspoon raw honey
- 1 teaspoon pure vanilla extract
- ¼ teaspoon salt
- 1 tablespoon coconut oil, divided

In a large mixing bowl, combine the hazelnut flour and blueberries. Toss them in the flour by hand. This keeps them from sinking to the bottom of the batter.

In a small bowl, beat together the eggs, almond milk, baking soda, honey, vanilla, and salt until blended, and then fold into flour–berry mixture. The batter will be lumpy; do not overmix. Let the batter stand for 10 minutes.

In a medium heavy skillet, melt a dime-size amount of the coconut oil over medium heat.

Ladle pancake batter into the skillet and make a 3- to 4-inch pancake. Cook the pancakes one or two at a time for 3 minutes on the first side, or until bubbles form at the edges, and then flip over and cook for 1 minute on the other side. As the pancakes are cooked, stack them on a plate and cover to keep warm.

Repeat with the remaining batter, adding more coconut oil to the skillet as needed.

To serve, stack a few pancakes on each plate and top with warm maple syrup or raw honey.

Serves 4.

Paleo Coconut Flour Pancakes

Coconut flour pancakes are delicate and lend themselves very well to fruit toppings or syrups. They're just as yummy paired with maple syrup.

- 1 cup coconut flour
- ½ cup toasted unsweetened coconut flakes
- 2 teaspoons baking soda
- ½ teaspoon salt
- 2 cups plain coconut milk
- 8 large eggs, beaten
- 2 teaspoons raw honey
- 1 teaspoon pure vanilla extract
- 1 tablespoon coconut oil, divided

In a large mixing bowl, combine the coconut flour, coconut flakes, baking soda, and salt, and mix well.

In a separate bowl, whisk together the coconut milk, eggs, honey, and vanilla until well blended. Fold the mixture into the dry ingredients and stir just until a lumpy batter forms. Set aside for 10 minutes.

In a medium heavy skillet, melt a dime-size amount of the coconut oil over medium heat.

Ladle pancake batter into the skillet and make a 3- to 4-inch pancake. Cook the pancakes one or two at a time for 3 minutes on the first side, or until bubbles form at the edges, and then flip over and cook for 1 minute on the other side. As the pancakes are cooked, stack them on a plate and cover to keep warm.

Repeat with the remaining batter, adding more coconut oil to the skillet as needed.

To serve, stack a few pancakes on each plate and top with warm maple syrup or fruit.

Serves 4.

Orange-Kissed Coconut Pancakes

Pictured on the book cover, these pancakes get a beautiful color and wonderfully bright taste from orange zest and a bit of orange juice concentrate. Top with the orange syrup for a plate full of sunshine that the whole family will love.

For the pancakes:
- 1 cup coconut flour
- 2 teaspoons baking soda
- 1 tablespoon orange zest
- ½ teaspoon salt
- 2 cups plain coconut milk
- 8 large eggs, beaten
- 2 tablespoons unsweetened orange juice concentrate, at room temperature
- 1 tablespoon coconut oil, divided

For the orange maple syrup:
- ½ cup maple syrup
- 2 teaspoons orange zest
- ½ teaspoon pure vanilla extract

To make the pancakes:

In a large mixing bowl, combine the coconut flour, baking soda, orange zest, and salt, and mix well.

In a separate bowl, whisk together the coconut milk, eggs, and orange juice concentrate, and stir until well blended. Fold the mixture into the dry ingredients and stir just until a lumpy batter forms. Set aside for 10 minutes.

In a medium heavy skillet, melt a dime-size amount of the coconut oil over medium heat.

Ladle pancake batter into the skillet and make a 3- to 4-inch pancake. Cook the pancakes one or two at a time for 3 minutes on the first side, or until bubbles form at the edges, and then flip over and cook for 1 minute on the other side. As the pancakes are cooked, stack them on a plate and cover to keep warm.

Repeat to cook the remaining batter, adding more coconut oil to the skillet as needed.

To make the orange maple syrup:

In a small saucepan, combine the maple syrup and orange zest, and cook over low heat for 5 minutes, stirring occasionally. Remove from the heat and stir in the vanilla. Keep warm.

To serve, stack a few pancakes on each plate and top with orange maple syrup.

Serves 4.

Paleo Grain-Free Banana Pancakes

The addition of mashed banana to grain-free pancakes not only adds great flavor, but just the right amount of moisture to keep them from being dry. Use overripe bananas for the most intense flavor.

- 2 cups hazelnut flour
- 1 teaspoon baking soda
- ¼ teaspoon salt
- 1 cup mashed ripe banana (about 2 large)
- 4 large eggs, beaten
- ½ cup plain almond milk
- 1 teaspoon pure vanilla extract
- 1 tablespoon coconut oil, divided

In a large mixing bowl, combine the hazelnut flour, baking soda, and salt. Add the banana and stir until well blended.

In a small bowl, whisk together the eggs, almond milk, and vanilla until blended. Fold the wet ingredients into flour mixture. The batter will be lumpy; do not overmix. Let the batter stand for 10 minutes.

In a medium heavy skillet, melt a dime-size amount of the coconut oil over medium heat.

Ladle pancake batter into the skillet and make a 3- to 4-inch pancake. Cook the pancakes one or two at a time for 3 minutes on the first side, or until bubbles form at the edges, and then flip over and cook for 1 minute on the other side. As the pancakes are cooked, stack them on a plate and cover to keep warm.

Repeat with the remaining batter, adding more coconut oil to the skillet as needed.

To serve, stack a few pancakes on each plate and top with warm maple syrup or raw honey.

Serves 4.

Mixed Berry Pancakes

These moist and beautiful pancakes are loaded with fresh berries. They're so good you may not even need syrup! Simply top with additional berries.

- 1 cup coconut flour
- 2 teaspoons baking soda
- ½ teaspoon salt
- 1 cup fresh berries (any combination of blueberries, strawberries, and blackberries)
- 2 cups plain coconut milk
- 8 large eggs, beaten
- 2 teaspoons raw honey
- 1 teaspoon pure vanilla extract
- 1 tablespoon coconut oil, divided

In a large mixing bowl, combine the coconut flour, baking soda, and salt, and mix well. Fold in the berries and toss by hand to coat with flour.

In a separate bowl, whisk together the coconut milk, eggs, honey, and vanilla until well blended. Fold the mixture into the dry ingredients and stir just until a lumpy batter forms. Set aside for 10 minutes.

In a medium heavy skillet, melt a dime-size amount of the coconut oil over medium heat.

Ladle pancake batter into the skillet and make a 3- to 4-inch pancake. Cook the pancakes one or two at a time for 3 minutes on the first side, or until bubbles form at the edges, and then flip over and cook for 1 minute on the other side. As the pancakes are cooked, stack them on a plate and cover to keep warm.

Repeat with remaining batter, adding more coconut oil to the skillet as needed.

To serve, stack a few pancakes on each plate and top with warm maple syrup or raw honey.

Serves 4.

Paleo Coconut Flour Waffles

This basic waffle recipe is great choice for the creative chef. Top with syrup or any fresh, seasonal fruit. For a delightful take on traditional syrup, see the orange maple syrup recipe earlier in this chapter.

- 1 cup coconut flour
- ½ cup tapioca flour
- 1 teaspoon baking soda
- ¼ teaspoon salt
- 4 large eggs, beaten
- ⅓ cup plain coconut milk
- 2 tablespoons coconut oil, melted
- 1 teaspoon pure vanilla extract

In a large mixing bowl, stir together the coconut and tapioca flours, baking soda, and salt until well blended.

In a separate bowl, mix together the eggs, coconut milk, coconut oil, and vanilla, then stir into the dry ingredients. Using a hand mixer, mix on low speed until well blended. Set aside for 10 minutes while heating the waffle iron.

Ladle batter into the waffle iron and cook according to manufacturer's instructions. As each waffle is finished, transfer it to a covered dish to keep warm.

Makes 4 waffles.

Paleo Banana Waffles

Mashed bananas make these waffles perfectly moist and sweet, and walnuts add some crunch. Think banana bread in a waffle iron! These freeze well, so make extra to reheat on other busy mornings.

- 1 cup coconut flour
- ½ cup tapioca flour
- 1 teaspoon baking soda
- ¼ teaspoon salt
- ½ cup chopped walnuts
- 4 large eggs, beaten
- ½ cup mashed ripe banana
- ¼ cup plain coconut milk
- 2 tablespoons coconut oil, melted
- 1 teaspoon pure vanilla extract

In a large mixing bowl, stir together the coconut and tapioca flours, baking soda, salt, and walnuts until well blended.

In a separate bowl, mix together the eggs, mashed banana, coconut milk, coconut oil, and vanilla, then stir into the dry ingredients. Using a hand mixer, mix on low speed until well blended. Set aside for 10 minutes while heating a waffle iron.

Ladle batter into the waffle iron and cook according to manufacturer's instructions. As each waffle is finished, transfer it to a covered dish to keep warm.

To serve, top the warm waffles with maple syrup or fruit.

Makes 4 waffles.

Hazelnut Waffles

Hazelnut flour and a hint of nutmeg give these waffles a distinct flavor that's a nice variation on regular waffles. Freeze a batch and pop them into the toaster when you're short on time in the morning.

- 1 cup hazelnut flour
- ½ cup tapioca flour
- 1 teaspoon baking soda
- ¼ teaspoon salt
- ½ teaspoon ground nutmeg
- ½ teaspoon ground cinnamon
- 4 large eggs, beaten
- ½ cup plain coconut milk
- 2 tablespoons coconut oil, melted
- 1 teaspoon pure vanilla extract

In a large mixing bowl, stir together the hazelnut and tapioca flours, baking soda, salt, nutmeg, and cinnamon until well blended.

In a separate bowl, mix together the eggs, coconut milk, coconut oil, and vanilla, then stir into the dry ingredients. Using a hand mixer, mix on low speed until well blended. Set aside for 10 minutes while heating a waffle iron.

Ladle batter into the waffle iron and cook according to manufacturer's instructions. As each waffle is finished, transfer it to a covered dish to keep warm.

To serve, top the warm waffles with maple syrup or fruit.

Makes 4 waffles.

9

PALEO EGGLESS BREAKFASTS

Chicken-Wrapped Asparagus Spears with Pine Nut Mayo

This dish is light and yet filling, and it's wonderful served with a Paleo muffin and some fresh fruit. To save time, you can flatten and cook the chicken breasts while you're fixing dinner the evening before.

For the chicken:
- 1 teaspoon olive oil
- 1 clove garlic, crushed
- 12 spears fresh asparagus, ends trimmed
- 4 small chicken breasts, pounded to ½-inch thickness
- ½ teaspoon salt
- ¼ teaspoon freshly ground black pepper

For the mayo:
- ½ cup raw pine nuts, soaked overnight and well drained
- ¼ cup water
- ½ lemon juiced and zested
- 1 pinch dry mustard (scant 1/8 teaspoon)
- 1 pinch kosher salt
- 2 tablespoons extra virgin olive oil
- 1 teaspoon apple cider vinegar

In a large heavy skillet, heat the olive oil over medium heat. Brown the garlic, add the asparagus, toss to coat with oil, and then spread into a single layer. Cover the pan and cook the asparagus, turning at least once, for 5 to 7 minutes, or until crisp-tender. Transfer to a plate.

Season the chicken breasts on both sides with the salt and pepper, and place them two at a time into the skillet. Increase to high heat and cook for about 3 minutes on each side, or until cooked through. Cook the remaining two breasts.

Place three asparagus spears onto each chicken breast, roll up, and secure with a toothpick. Cover to keep warm.

To make the mayo:
Combine all ingredients in a blender and process until smooth. Place 1/2 cup of the mayo in a small saucepan over medium head, stirring frequently until hot. Leftover mayo will keep for 1 week refrigerated.

To serve, place a chicken breast on each plate and drizzle with sauce.

Serves 4.

Paleo Hash

Traditional hash is made with corned or roast beef and white potatoes, but there are many delicious ways to prepare a savory breakfast hash. This recipe uses finely cubed sweet potatoes, bacon, and onions. It's wonderful.

- 6 slices unsmoked bacon or pancetta, chopped
- 2 medium sweet potatoes, peeled and finely diced
- 1 medium yellow onion, diced
- ½ teaspoon dried rosemary
- ½ teaspoon ground nutmeg
- ½ teaspoon freshly ground black pepper

In a large heavy skillet over medium-high heat, cook the bacon until it is well browned, 6 to 7 minutes.

Use a slotted spoon to transfer the bacon to a paper towel, and drain the skillet of all but 1 teaspoon of drippings.

Reduce the heat to medium and add the sweet potatoes and onions to the skillet. Sprinkle with the rosemary, nutmeg, and pepper, and sauté for about 10 minutes, or until the sweet potatoes have caramelized and are fork-tender. Stir in the bacon and heat through.

Serves 2 as an entrée or 4 as a side dish.

Sautéed Chicken Livers

Chicken livers are inexpensive and packed with flavor. This recipe is great served over toast, on Paleo-friendly crackers, or used as filling for deviled eggs.

- 1 pound well-drained chicken livers
- 2 teaspoons olive oil
- 4 cloves garlic, crushed
- 1 small yellow onion, chopped (about ½ cup)
- ½ teaspoon dried rosemary
- ½ teaspoon paprika
- ½ teaspoon salt
- ¼ teaspoon freshly ground black pepper

Place the chicken livers on a plate lined with paper towels and top with another paper towel. Gently press down to squeeze out any excess liquid, and allow the livers to sit for about 10 minutes before patting dry with another paper towel.

In a large heavy skillet, heat the olive oil over medium heat. Sauté the garlic and onion for 3 to 4 minutes, or until the onions are fairly tender, taking care not to let the garlic burn.

Add the livers, rosemary, paprika, salt, and pepper to the skillet, and increase the heat to medium-high. Sauté for 5 to 6 minutes, stirring frequently, until the largest piece of liver is cooked through.

Use a slotted spoon to transfer the livers to a platter, and serve warm.

Serves 4 to 6.

Chicken and Mushroom Wraps

Chicken breasts don't need to be relegated to lunch or dinner fare—they're equally good for breakfast. These are contained neatly in a lettuce leaf and can be wrapped in wax paper if you need something on the go.

- 1 teaspoon olive oil
- 2 chicken breasts (about ¾ pound), sliced into 1-inch pieces
- ½ teaspoon ground turmeric
- ½ teaspoon salt, divided
- ¼ cup chopped red onion
- ½ pound sliced fresh mushrooms
- ¼ cup chopped fresh parsley
- ½ teaspoon freshly ground black pepper
- 8 large leaves romaine lettuce

In a large heavy skillet, heat the olive oil over medium-high heat.

Sprinkle the chicken slices with the turmeric and ¼ teaspoon of the salt. Put in the skillet and sauté for 5 minutes on one side. Turn the slices over and add the onion, mushrooms, parsley, pepper, and the remaining ¼ teaspoon salt to the skillet. Sauté for 5 minutes, stirring frequently.

Meanwhile, lay two pieces of lettuce lengthwise, overlapping one another halfway, with the widest end closest to you.

Place a quarter of the chicken filling on the widest part of the lettuce leaves and carefully roll up going away from you. After one full roll, tuck the ends in burrito style before wrapping the rest of the way. If desired, roll in wax paper in the same fashion before cutting in half.

Repeat with the remaining lettuce and filling and serve.

Serves 4.

Paleo Sausage Gravy

Traditional Southern sausage gravy is made with white flour, but this recipe is adapted to the Paleo diet and uses Paleo-friendly sausage. Serve over scrambled eggs, Paleo toast, or your favorite Paleo muffin.

- 1 pound nitrate-free sausage
- 2 tablespoons almond flour
- 2 cups plain almond milk
- Salt and pepper to taste

In a large heavy skillet, brown the sausage over medium-high heat, stirring frequently to break it up, for about 6 minutes, or until cooked through.

Drain all but about 2 tablespoons of drippings, increase the heat to high, and quickly whisk in the almond flour. It should become pasty.

Slowly stir in the almond milk, scraping up the browned bits from the skillet. Reduce the heat to medium and cook, stirring frequently, for 3 to 4 minutes, or until the gravy has thickened. Taste for seasoning and add salt and pepper as needed.

To serve, ladle over Paleo-friendly toast or muffins, or use as a topping for scrambled eggs.

Serves 4.

Toast with Mushroom Sauce

This breakfast dish is creamy and comforting—a delicious way to start a chilly morning. You can make the mushroom sauce ahead of time, or even prepare a double batch and use the extra portion to top chicken breasts or scrambled eggs.

- 2 teaspoons olive oil
- ¼ cup chopped yellow onion
- 1 pound sliced white mushrooms
- 1 tablespoon chopped fresh tarragon, or 1 teaspoon dried
- 2 tablespoons chopped fresh parsley, plus additional for garnish
- ½ teaspoon salt
- ¼ teaspoon freshly ground black pepper
- 1 cup plain almond milk
- 4 slices thick Paleo-friendly bread, toasted

In a large heavy skillet, heat the olive oil over medium-high heat. Sauté the onion, mushrooms, tarragon, parsley, salt, and pepper for about 6 minutes, stirring frequently, until the mushrooms are slightly browned.

Stir in the almond milk, scraping up any browned bits from the skillet. Reduce the heat to medium, and cook for about 10 minutes, or until the sauce is slightly reduced and thickened. Remove from the heat and cover to keep warm.

To serve, place a piece of toast on each plate and ladle a quarter of the mushroom sauce on top. Garnish with additional parsley, if desired.

Serves 4.

Paleo Crab Cakes

In some European coastal communities and the Deep South, it is common to have fish and seafood for breakfast. This is an excellent way to get your feet wet if you've never had a little seafood in the morning.

- 1 teaspoon light olive oil
- ¼ cup finely chopped yellow onion
- 1 stalk celery, very finely chopped
- 12 ounces canned crabmeat, picked clean of any shell or cartilage
- 2 tablespoons pine nut mayo (see the first recipe in this chapter)
- ¼ teaspoon hot sauce
- ½ teaspoon dry mustard
- ½ teaspoon salt
- ½ teaspoon freshly ground black pepper

In a medium heavy skillet, heat the olive oil over medium-high heat. Sauté the onion and celery for 5 minutes, just until the celery is fairly tender. Transfer to a bowl and let cool to room temperature.

In a mixing bowl, stir together the crabmeat, pine nut mayo, hot sauce, dry mustard, salt, and pepper, and mix well. Fold in the celery and onions.

Return the skillet to medium-high heat, and pat the crab mixture into four cakes about 1½ inches thick. Cook for about 4 minutes on each side, or until the cakes are golden.

To serve, place a crab cake on each plate and serve with fresh fruit and a Paleo muffin.

Serves 4.

Sausage-Stuffed Portobello Mushrooms

This recipe is quick and easy and uses only one skillet, which is a plus on busy mornings. While these stuffed mushrooms are great for breakfast, they are equally good as a lunch dish or a side dish at dinner. They reheat well, so you can make extra and they'll keep in the fridge for about 3 days.

- ½ pound nitrate-free sausage
- ½ cup chopped yellow onion
- 4 large whole portobello mushrooms
- 1 cup fresh baby spinach leaves
- ½ teaspoon paprika
- ½ teaspoon salt
- ¼ teaspoon freshly ground black pepper

In a large heavy skillet, brown the sausage over medium-high heat for 5 minutes, stirring frequently to break it up as it cooks. Stir in the onion.

Trim the stems from the mushrooms and chop roughly, and then add to the skillet. Add the spinach, paprika, salt, and pepper, and cook for 5 minutes, or until the sausage is cooked through.

Divide the filling between the mushroom caps. Place the mushrooms in the skillet, cover the pan, and reduce the heat to medium. Cook for 5 minutes or until the mushrooms are tender and nicely browned.

To serve, place a stuffed mushroom on each plate and serve with a salad or fresh fruit.

Serves 4.

Turkey Steaks with Fried Apples

This recipe makes delicious use of leftover turkey breast. With the aromatic fried apples, it's a wonderful way to start a cool autumn morning.

- 1 teaspoon coconut oil
- 4 firm apples (such as Gala or Golden Delicious), cored and sliced
- 1 teaspoon ground cinnamon
- ½ teaspoon ground nutmeg
- ½ teaspoon salt
- ¼ teaspoon freshly ground black pepper
- 2 thick slices (about 6 ounces) cooked turkey breast

In a large heavy skillet, heat the coconut oil over medium heat.

In a mixing bowl, sprinkle the apples with the cinnamon, nutmeg, salt, and pepper, and toss to coat.

Add the apples to the skillet and sauté, stirring every so often, for about 10 minutes, or until nearly tender.

Place the turkey slices in the center of the skillet, cover with some of the apple slices, and cover the pan. Cook for an additional 5 minutes, or until the turkey is heated through.

To serve, place a slice of turkey on each plate and top with half of the apples.

Serves 2.

10

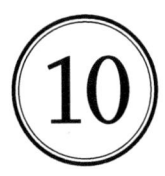

PALEO BREAKFAST BARS

Sweet Potato Breakfast Bars

These bars are moist and flavorful, and they come with all the fiber and beta-carotene that sweet potatoes provide. They don't freeze well but will keep for 1 week in an airtight container.

- ½ teaspoon coconut oil
- 2 large baked sweet potatoes
- 3 tablespoons almond flour
- 1 cup unsweetened coconut flakes
- ¼ teaspoon baking soda
- ¼ teaspoon cream of tartar
- ½ teaspoon ground cinnamon
- ¼ teaspoon salt
- ¼ teaspoon ground nutmeg
- 1 cup unsweetened golden raisins
- ¼ cup coconut oil, melted
- ½ cup raw honey

Preheat the oven to 350 degrees F. Grease a 9 x 13 inch baking pan with the coconut oil and set aside.

Split open the sweet potatoes and spoon the flesh into a large mixing bowl. Use a fork or hand mixer to mash the potatoes until smooth.

Stir in the almond flour, coconut flakes, baking soda, and cream of tartar until well combined, then add the cinnamon, salt, and nutmeg, and mix well. Add the raisins, melted coconut oil, and honey, stirring to incorporate.

Transfer the batter to the baking pan and smooth it into an even layer. Bake for 35 to 40 minutes, or until a toothpick inserted into the center comes out clean. Let cool for 1 hour before cutting into bars.

Makes 1 dozen bars.

Banana-Pecan Bars

These breakfast bars will remind you of homemade banana bread. They freeze very well wrapped in plastic wrap and then aluminum foil, so plan to make extra to keep on hand.

- 1 teaspoon coconut oil
- 6 large very ripe bananas, mashed
- 2 large eggs, beaten
- ½ cup coconut oil, melted
- 1 teaspoon pure vanilla extract
- 1 cup coconut flour
- 1 teaspoon baking soda
- ½ teaspoon ground nutmeg
- ½ teaspoon ground cinnamon
- ¼ teaspoon salt
- 1 cup raisins
- ¾ cup chopped pecans

Preheat the oven to 375 degrees F. Grease a 9 x 13 inch baking pan with the coconut oil and set aside.

In a large mixing bowl, combine the bananas, eggs, melted coconut oil, and vanilla. Beat on low speed for about 1 minute, just until blended. Add the coconut flour, baking soda, nutmeg, cinnamon, and salt, and beat for 1 to 2 minutes, or until the ingredients are well blended. Add the raisins and pecans, stirring to incorporate.

Transfer the batter to the baking pan and smooth it into an even layer. Bake for 35 to 40 minutes, or until a toothpick inserted into the center comes out clean.

Let cool to room temperature before cutting into bars. Store the bars wrapped in plastic wrap in the fridge for up to 1 week. To freeze, wrap in plastic wrap and then aluminum foil, and store in the freezer for up to 6 months.

Makes 1 dozen bars.

Applesauce-Raisin Bars

Applesauce contributes wonderful moistness to these bars. Walnuts add the crunch and raisins add another hint of chewy sweetness. These bars go very fast but freeze well, so double the batch!

- 1 teaspoon coconut oil
- 2 cups unsweetened applesauce
- 2 large eggs, beaten
- ½ cup coconut oil, melted
- 1 teaspoon pure vanilla extract
- 1 cup coconut flour
- 1 teaspoon baking soda
- ½ teaspoon ground allspice
- ¼ teaspoon salt
- 1 cup unsweetened raisins
- ¾ cup chopped walnuts

Preheat the oven to 375 degrees F. Grease a 9 x 13 inch pan with the coconut oil and set aside.

In a large mixing bowl, combine the applesauce, eggs, melted coconut oil, and vanilla. Beat on low speed for about 1 minute, until well blended. Add the coconut flour, baking soda, allspice, and salt, and beat for 1 to 2 minutes, or until the ingredients are well blended. Add the raisins, stirring to incorporate.

Transfer the batter to the baking pan and smooth it into an even layer. Sprinkle the chopped walnuts over the top. Bake for 35 to 40 minutes, or until a toothpick inserted into the center comes out clean.

Let cool to room temperature before cutting into bars. Store the bars wrapped in plastic wrap in the fridge for up to 1 week. To freeze, wrap in plastic wrap and then aluminum foil, and store in the freezer for up to 6 months.

Makes 1 dozen bars.

Paleo Pumpkin Bars

If your family likes pumpkin pie, they'll love these fantastic bars. For an added treat, serve warm topped with a little bit of maple syrup. They freeze very well, so make a double batch.

- 1 teaspoon coconut oil
- 1 (28-ounce) can pumpkin puree (not pumpkin pie filling)
- 2 large eggs, beaten
- 1 tablespoon coconut oil, melted
- 1 teaspoon pure vanilla extract
- 1 cup almond flour
- 1 teaspoon ground cinnamon
- ½ teaspoon ground ginger
- ½ teaspoon ground allspice
- 1 teaspoon baking soda
- 1 cup chopped walnuts

Preheat the oven to 350 degrees F. Grease a 9 x 13 inch baking pan with the coconut oil and set aside.

In a large bowl, combine the pumpkin puree, eggs, melted coconut oil, and vanilla, and stir until well blended.

In a separate bowl, combine the almond flour, cinnamon, ginger, allspice, and baking soda. Stir together until well blended. Fold the dry ingredients into the pumpkin mixture, stirring just until blended.

Transfer the batter to the baking pan and smooth it into an even layer. Sprinkle the chopped walnuts over the top. Bake for 45 to 50 minutes, or until a toothpick inserted in the center comes out clean. Let cool to room temperature before cutting into bars.

Makes 1 dozen bars.

Fruity Coconut Bars

These bars are chewy, sweet, and a big hit with kids. Have them for breakfast, pack them in lunch bags, or enjoy them as an evening snack.

- 1 teaspoon coconut oil
- 6 large very ripe bananas, mashed
- 2 eggs, beaten
- ½ cup coconut oil, melted
- 1 teaspoon pure vanilla extract
- 1 cup coconut flour
- 1 teaspoon baking soda
- ½ teaspoon ground nutmeg
- ¼ teaspoon salt
- 1 cup unsweetened coconut flakes
- 1 cup chopped dried apricots

Preheat the oven to 375 degrees F. Grease a 9 x 13 inch baking pan with the coconut oil and set aside.

In a large mixing bowl, combine the bananas, eggs, melted coconut oil, and vanilla. Beat on low speed for about 1 minute, until well blended. Add the coconut flour, baking soda, nutmeg, and salt, and beat for 1 to 2 minutes, or until all the ingredients are well blended. Add the coconut flakes and apricots, stirring to incorporate.

Transfer the batter to the baking pan and smooth it into an even layer. Bake for 35 to 40 minutes, or until a toothpick inserted into the center comes out clean.

Let cool to room temperature before cutting into bars. Store the bars wrapped in plastic wrap in the fridge for up to 1 week. To freeze, wrap in plastic wrap and then aluminum foil, and store in the freezer for up to 6 months.

Makes 1 dozen bars.

Coconut-Almond Bars

These bars are chock-full of nuts, coconut, and creamy almond butter. They not only are great for breakfast but make a terrific post-workout snack or lunch box treat.

- 1 teaspoon coconut oil
- 1 cup unsweetened applesauce
- 1 cup almond butter
- 2 eggs, beaten
- ½ cup coconut oil, melted
- 1 teaspoon pure vanilla extract
- 1½ cups almond flour
- 1 teaspoon baking soda
- ½ teaspoon ground nutmeg
- ½ teaspoon ground cinnamon
- ¼ teaspoon salt
- 1 cup unsweetened coconut flakes
- 1 cup chopped almonds

Preheat the oven to 375 degrees F. Grease a 9 x 13 inch baking pan with the coconut oil and set aside.

In a large mixing bowl, combine the applesauce, almond butter, melted coconut oil, and vanilla. Beat on low speed for about 1 minute, until well blended. Add the almond flour, baking soda, nutmeg, cinnamon, and salt, and beat for 1 to 2 minutes, or until the ingredients are well blended. Add the coconut flakes and almonds, stirring to incorporate.

Transfer the batter to the baking pan and smooth it into an even layer. Bake for 35 to 40 minutes, or until a toothpick inserted into the center comes out clean.

Let cool to room temperature before cutting into bars. Store the bars wrapped in plastic wrap in the fridge for up to 1 week. To freeze, wrap in plastic wrap and then aluminum foil, and store in the freezer for up to 6 months.

Makes 1 dozen bars.

Hazelnut-Peach Breakfast Bars

These breakfast bars get their natural sweetness from applesauce and fresh peaches. As they bake, their aroma will perfume your house.

- 1 teaspoon coconut oil
- 1½ cups unsweetened applesauce
- ½ cup plain almond milk
- 2 large eggs, beaten
- ½ cup coconut oil, melted
- 1 teaspoon pure vanilla extract
- 1 cup hazelnut flour
- 1 teaspoon baking soda
- ½ teaspoon ground nutmeg
- ¼ teaspoon salt
- 6 large fresh peaches, sliced
- ½ cup slivered almonds

Preheat the oven to 375 degrees F. Grease a 9 x 13 inch baking pan with the coconut oil and set aside.

In a large mixing bowl, combine the applesauce, almond milk, eggs, melted coconut oil, and vanilla. Beat on low speed for about 1 minute, until well blended.

In a separate bowl, combine the hazelnut flour, baking soda, nutmeg, and salt, and then add to the wet ingredients, stirring with a wooden spoon until well incorporated.

Transfer the batter to the baking pan and smooth it into an even layer. Arrange the peach slices over the top in a nice pattern, pressing down just a bit so that the peaches are half submerged in the batter. Sprinkle the slivered almonds on top.

Bake for 45 to 50 minutes, or until a toothpick inserted into the center comes out clean. Let cool to room temperature before cutting into bars.

Makes 1 dozen bars.

Paleo Granola Bars

This recipe is far better for you than any commercial granola bars, which are often laden with high-fructose corn syrup and unhealthy grains. They bake up in a jiffy and will keep in an airtight container for up to 1 week—that is, if they last that long.

- 1 teaspoon coconut oil
- 1 cup pecan pieces
- 1 cup pumpkin seeds
- 1 cup chopped walnuts
- 1 cup dried cranberries
- 1 cup dried apricots, chopped
- 1 cup unsweetened coconut flakes
- ¼ cup coconut oil, melted
- ½ cup almond butter
- ½ cup raw honey
- ¼ teaspoon pure vanilla extract
- ½ teaspoon salt
- 1 teaspoon ground cinnamon

Preheat the oven to 325 degrees F. Grease a 9 x 13 inch baking pan with the coconut oil and set aside.

In a large bowl, combine the pecans, pumpkin seeds, walnuts, cranberries, apricots, and coconut flakes, and toss to mix well.

In a small saucepan over low heat, combine the melted coconut oil, almond butter, honey, vanilla, salt, and cinnamon, and heat just until the honey is completely melted.

Transfer the nut mixture to the baking pan, pressing down to spread it evenly. Pour the oil-honey mixture evenly over the top.

Bake for 35 to 40 minutes, or until golden. Let cool to room temperature before cutting into bars. Store in an airtight container for up to 1 week.

Makes 1 dozen bars.

No-Bake Fruit and Nut Bars

There are few snacks as beloved as chewy snack bars, and these make the perfect on-the-go breakfast. These ones hit all the right notes, with a combination of nuts, coconut, honey, and dried fruit. As a bonus, you don't even have to bake to enjoy these treats! The bars keep well, so make several batches at once.

- 2 cups raw pecan halves or pieces
- 2 cups raw walnut halves or pieces
- ½ teaspoon sea salt
- ½ teaspoon cinnamon
- ¼ teaspoon nutmeg
- 3 tablespoons plus ½ teaspoon coconut oil, melted
- ½ cup unsweetened shredded coconut
- ½ cup dried, unsweetened cranberries, chopped
- ½ cup dried, unsweetened cherries, chopped
- ½ cup raw honey

In a food processor or blender, grind the pecans and walnuts together until they are similar to breadcrumbs in consistency. Work in batches and be careful not to grind them too long or you will end up with pecan-walnut butter!

Pour the ground nuts into a large mixing bowl and add salt, cinnamon, and nutmeg, mixing well with your hands or a large spoon. Pour 3 tablespoons coconut oil over the mixture and blend well.

Stir in the shredded coconut, cranberries, and cherries until well mixed, then add the honey. Line a 9 x 13 inch baking pan with aluminum foil and lightly grease the bottom and sides with ½ teaspoon coconut oil. Use a spoon or sturdy spatula to spread the mixture evenly into the baking pan, pressing it down firmly.

Cover with foil and let sit for 3–4 hours before cutting into bars.

Store in an airtight container for up to 1 week, or you can freeze them for up to 3 months.

Makes 1 dozen bars.

11

LIVING ON THE PALEO DIET

What Is the Paleo Diet?

The Paleo diet is a pretty dramatic departure from the typical Western diet. Although there are several versions of the Paleo diet, all are based on the same basic principle: eating a diet more like that of our ancient ancestors, which means excluding processed foods, grains, legumes, dairy, refined sugars, and most alcoholic beverages.

The premise behind the Paleo diet is that we are not genetically programmed to process foods such as legumes, grains, and dairy, and that many of the health problems we have today are a result of eating foods to which our bodies are not truly adapted.

These health issues—such as obesity, diabetes, and heart disease—are often referred to as "diseases of affluence." This is because they are most common, and even considered epidemic, in the wealthier nations, where people eat rich diets far removed from the land. The typical Western diet is filled with starchy and sugar-dense carbohydrates such as breads, cereals, and cakes; large quantity of dairy products; and highly processed and packaged foods. Many of these foods are high in sugar, unhealthy fats, and empty calories, but are very low in nutrition.

The creators of the various versions of the Paleo diet claim that many nutrition-related diseases can be avoided or reversed by following the Paleo pattern of eating. A good deal of research supports this claim. As a side benefit, the Paleo diet can also help followers to lose weight, although its main purpose is improved health, specifically, good cardiovascular health and a stronger immune system.

Many people have expressed concern that a diet that was meat-centric had to be unhealthful for the heart and arteries, but several studies have shown that the Paleo guideline of eating grass-fed organic meats is very healthful indeed. A 2009 research study conducted by Clemson University and the U.S. Department of Agriculture showed that compared to feedlot meats, grass-fed meats are higher in antioxidants, vitamins, and minerals; lower in the saturated fats associated with heart disease; lower in total fat; and higher in CLA (conjugated linoleic acid), which is thought to fight some types of cancers. It also has a higher amount of omega-3 fatty acids and a healthier ratio of omega-3 to omega-6 fats.

Many people report feeling "lighter" and more energetic on the Paleo diet, and it has become very popular with athletes as well as those who want a healthy way to lose weight without going hungry.

What Does It Mean to Eat Gluten-Free?

Eating gluten-free isn't just about cutting wheat from your diet. Gluten is also found in cereal grains such as rye, barley, oats, and many others. Many people unfamiliar with a gluten-free diet believe that it means going without any kind of bread, crackers, muffins, cakes, cookies, or other baked goods. Happily, this couldn't be further from the truth.

While flours made from wheat, rye, barley, oats, and other cereal grains are most commonly used in making breads and other baked goods, there are a great variety of other flours from which to choose. Nut flours like almond, coconut, and hazelnut are some of the most commonly used alternatives in the Paleo diet.

The consumption of grains, dairy products, and legumes is being blamed more and more for the increase in immune disorders and symptoms of immune system imbalances. Many studies support this theory. In 2011, Dr. Jean Seignalet conducted a study of several hundred patients with various immune disorders who were put on a Paleo diet. One hundred percent of the lupus patients showed at least a 50 percent improvement in their symptoms, as did 97 percent of patients with fibromyalgia and multiple sclerosis.

Many studies have shown that just a couple of weeks on a gluten-free diet shows remarkable improvement with gluten-related symptoms such as bloating, gas, loose bowels, inflammation, and fatigue. It's nice to know that those few weeks don't have to mean living without dinner rolls and blueberry muffins.

A truly gluten-free diet that is prescribed for those diagnosed with celiac disease excludes not just grain products but some types of vitamins, condiments, beverages, and other items that are made using gluten as a filler or stabilizer. Unless you are diagnosed with celiac disease or a serious gluten-sensitivity, you don't need to go to such extremes. However, you'll likely see many other benefits from the lack of gluten in your food when you adopt the Paleo diet.

Note: If you suspect that you may have celiac disease, it's very important that you don't go on a gluten-free diet before being tested. According to Dr. Stefano Guandalini, founder of the University of Chicago Celiac Disease Center, just a few weeks without gluten can skew test results for celiac, as they're based on the presence of antibodies. (Hill ID, et al.; *North American Society for Pediatric Gastroenterology, Hepatology, and Nutrition*, 2005 Jan.; 40(1):1–19.)

Cutting grains from your diet may seem daunting at first, but the delicious recipes in this book, coupled with how much better you'll feel on the Paleo diet, will make you forget all about those grain-based foods you think you'll miss.

The Paleo Diet Foods List

Meats and Seafood

Meats

- Lean beef (trimmed of visible fat)
    - Flank steak
    - Top sirloin steak
    - Extra lean hamburger (7% fat or less)
    - London broil
    - Lean veal
    - Chuck steak
    - Any other lean cut of beef
- Lean pork (trimmed of visible fat)
    - Pork loin
    - Pork chops
    - Any other lean cut of pork
- Lean poultry (white meat, skin removed)

- Chicken breast
- Turkey breast
- Game hen breasts
- Eggs (Although many diets recommend only eating the whites, whole eggs are recommended for the Paleo diet. You can have eggs from chickens, ducks, or geese. Do not buy egg substitutes.)
- Rabbit meat (any cut)
- Goat meat (any cut)
- Organ meats
  - Beef, lamb, pork, and chicken livers and kidneys
  - Chicken or turkey gizzards and hearts
  - Beef, lamb, and pork tongues
  - Beef, lamb, and pork marrow
  - Beef, lamb, and pork sweetbreads
- Game meats
  - Alligator
  - Bear
  - Bison (buffalo)
  - Caribou
  - Elk
  - Emu
  - Goose
  - Kangaroo
  - Muscovy duck
  - New Zealand Cervena deer
  - Ostrich
  - Pheasant
  - Quail
  - Rattlesnake
  - Reindeer
  - Squab
  - Turtle
  - Venison
  - Wild boar
  - Wild turkey

Seafood

- Abalone
- Bass
- Bluefish
- Branzini (Mediterranean sea bass)
- Clams
- Cod
- Crab
- Crayfish
- Drum
- Eel
- Flatfish
- Grouper
- Haddock
- Halibut
- Herring
- Lobster
- Mackerel
- Monkfish
- Mullet
- Mussels
- Northern pike
- Orange roughy
- Oysters
- Perch
- Red snapper
- Rockfish
- Salmon (fillet, steak, patties, or smoked)
- Sardines
- Scallops
- Scrod (a young cod weighing 2½ pounds or less)
- Shark

- Shrimp
- Striped bass
- Sunfish
- Swordfish
- Tilapia
- Trout
- Tuna
- Turbot
- Walleye
- Any other commercially available fish

Fruits and Vegetables

Fruits

- Apple
- Apricot
- Avocado
- Banana
- Blackberries
- Blueberries
- Boysenberries
- Cantaloupe
- Cherries
- Cherimoya
- Cranberries
- Gooseberries
- Grapefruit
- Grapes
- Guava
- Honeydew melon

- Kiwi
- Lemon
- Lime
- Lychee
- Mango
- Nectarine
- Orange
- Papaya
- Passion fruit
- Peach
- Pear
- Persimmon
- Pineapple
- Plum
- Pomegranate
- Raspberries
- Rhubarb
- Star fruit (Carambola)
- Tangerine
- Watermelon
- All other fruits

Vegetables

- Artichoke
- Asparagus
- Beet greens
- Beets
- Bell peppers
- Broccoli
- Brussels sprouts
- Cabbage
- Carrots

- Cauliflower
- Celery
- Collard greens
- Cucumber
- Dandelion greens
- Eggplant
- Endive
- Green onions
- Kale
- Kohlrabi
- Lettuce (except iceberg)
- Mushrooms
- Mustard greens
- Onions
- Parsley
- Parsnip
- Peppers (all kinds)
- Pumpkin
- Purslane
- Radish
- Rutabaga
- Seaweed
- Spinach
- Squash (all kinds)
- Swiss chard
- Tomatillos
- Tomatoes
- Turnip greens
- Turnips
- Watercress
- Zucchini

Nuts, Seeds, and Oils

- Almond butter
- Almonds
- Brazil nuts
- Cashews
- Chestnuts
- Coconut oil
- Flaxseed
- Hazelnuts
- Macadamia nuts
- Nut flours (almond, coconut, or hazelnut is recommended)
- Olive oil
- Palm oil
- Pecans
- Pine nuts
- Pistachios
- Pumpkin seeds
- Sesame butter or tahini (pure, raw)
- Sesame seeds
- Sunflower seeds
- Walnuts

Beverages

- Water
- Green tea
- Herbal tea
- Moderate amounts of organic pure fruit juice without added sugar

Other

- Fresh and dried herbs
- Spices and seasonings
- Frozen fruits and fruit bars without added sugar
- Dried fruits without added sugar
- Carob powder
- Organic raw honey

Foods to Avoid on the Paleo Diet

Dairy

- All foods made with any dairy products
- Butter
- Cheese
- Dairy spreads
- Frozen yogurt
- Ice cream
- Ice milk
- Low-fat milk
- Nonfat dairy creamer
- Powdered milk
- Skim milk
- Whole milk
- Yogurt

Cereal Grains

- Amaranth
- Barley
    - barley soup

- - barley bread
  - barley malt
  - pearl barley
  - all processed foods made with barley
- Buckwheat
- Corn
  - corn on the cob
  - corn tortillas
  - corn chips
  - cornstarch
  - corn syrup
- Couscous
- Farina
- Millet
- Oats
  - steel-cut oats
  - rolled oats
  - all processed foods made with oats
- Rice
  - brown rice
  - white rice
  - rice noodles
  - basmati rice
  - rice cakes
  - rice flour
  - all processed foods made with rice
- Rye
  - rye bread
  - rye crackers
  - all processed foods made with rye
- Semolina
- Sorghum

- Wheat
    - bread, rolls
    - muffins
    - noodles
    - crackers
    - cookies
    - doughnuts
    - pancakes
    - waffles
    - pasta
    - spaghetti
    - lasagna
    - wheat tortillas
    - pizza
    - pita bread
    - flat bread
    - all processed foods made with wheat or wheat flour

Legumes

- Beans
    - adzuki beans
    - black beans
    - broad beans
    - fava beans
    - field beans
    - garbanzo beans
    - horse beans
    - kidney beans
    - lima beans
    - mung beans
    - navy beans
    - pinto beans

- - red beans
  - string beans
  - white beans
- Black-eyed peas
- Chickpeas
- Lentils
- Peanuts and peanut butter
- Peas
- Snow peas
- Soybeans
  - edamame
  - soy milk
  - tofu
- Sugar snap peas

Starchy Vegetables

- Cassava root
- Manioc
- Potatoes and all potato products (such as French fries and potato chips)
- Tapioca
- Yams

High-Salt Meats, Snacks, and Sauces

- Bacon (use the lean portions occasionally for seasoning/cooking)
- Deli meats
- Hot dogs
- Ketchup
- Kielbasa or smoked sausage
- Nearly all canned meats or and fish
- Pickled foods
- Pork rinds

- Processed meats
- Salami
- Salted nuts
- Salted spices
- Sausages
- Smoked, dried and salted fish and meat
- Teriyaki sauce

Other

- Alcohol
  - beer (note that gluten-free beers are available)
  - bourbon
  - Scotch
  - vodka
- Malted vinegars

Foods that Require Caution

The following items may or may not contain gluten, depending on where and how they are made. It is sometimes necessary to check with the manufacturer to find out.

- Artificial color[3]
- Baking powder[3]
- Caramel color[1,2]
- Caramel flavoring[1,2]
- Clarifying agents[3]
- Coloring[3]
- Dextrimaltose[1]
- Dextrins[1]
- Dry-roasted nuts[3]
- Emulsifiers[3]
- Enzymes[3]
- Fat replacer[3]

- Flavoring[5]
- Food starch modified[1,3]
- Food starch[1,3]
- Glucose syrup[3]
- Gravy cubes[3]
- Ground spices[3]
- HPP[4]
- HVP[4]
- Hydrogenated starch hydrolysate[3]
- Hydrolyzed plant protein[3]
- Hydrolyzed protein[3]
- Hydrolyzed vegetable protein[3]
- Hydroxy-propylated starch[3]
- Maltose[3]
- Miso[3]
- Mixed tocopherols[3]
- Modified food starch[1,3]
- Modified starch[1,3]
- Natural flavoring[5]
- Natural flavors[5]
- Natural juices[3]
- Non-dairy creamer[3]
- Pre-gelatinized starch[3]
- Protein hydrolysates[3]
- Seafood analogs[3]
- Seasonings[3]
- Sirimi[3]
- Smoke flavoring[3]
- Soba noodles[3]
- Soy sauce solids[3]
- Soy sauce[3]
- Sphingolipids[3]
- Stabilizers[3]

- Starch[1,3]
- Stock cubes[3]
- Suet[4]
- Tocopherols[3]
- Vegetable broth[3]
- Vegetable gum[3]
- Vegetable protein[3]
- Vegetable starch[3]
- Vitamins[3]
- Wheat starch[4]

---

[1]. If this ingredient is made in North America, it is likely to be gluten-free.

[2]. The problem with caramel color is it may or may not contain gluten, depending on how it is manufactured. In the United States, caramel color must conform to FDA standards, as outlined in the Code of Federal Regulations Title 21 (21 CFR), Part 73. This regulation states: "The color additive caramel is the dark-brown liquid or solid material resulting from the carefully controlled heat treatment of the following food-grade carbohydrates: Dextrose [corn sugar], invert sugar, lactose [milk sugar], malt syrup [usually from barley malt], molasses [from sugar cane], starch hydrolysates and fractions thereof [which can include wheat], sucrose [cane or beet sugar]."

[3]. May use a grain or byproduct containing gluten in the manufacturing process, or as an ingredient.

[4]. Most celiac disease support organizations in the United States and Canada do not believe that wheat starch is safe for people with celiac disease. In Europe, however, most doctors and celiac disease support organizations consider Codex Alimentarius Quality wheat starch acceptable in the celiac diet. This is a higher quality of wheat starch than is generally available in the United States or Canada.

[5]. According to 21 CFR, Section 101.22: "The term natural flavor or natural flavoring means the essential oil, oleoresin, essence or extractive, protein hydrolysate, distillate, or any product of roasting, heating or enzymolysis, which contains the flavoring constituents derived from a spice, fruit or fruit juice, vegetable or vegetable juice, edible yeast, herb, bark, bud, root, leaf or similar plant material, meat, seafood, poultry, eggs, dairy products, or fermentation products thereof, whose significant function in food is flavoring rather than nutritional."

CONCLUSION

We all want to live longer, feel better, and look fit and healthy, but few of us are willing to live life feeling deprived in order to do it.

The Paleo diet allows you to eat plenty of delicious whole foods; you don't have to count calories, and you can enjoy lots of treats and snacks that will keep you from feeling like you're missing out. The Paleo diet isn't about weight loss as much as it is about optimal health, but many people find that they lose weight on the diet.

More important, most people report that they feel wonderful after just a couple of weeks without processed foods, grains, sugar, and unhealthy fats. This is the greatest benefit of the diet, because there really isn't much point in losing weight if you don't feel up to enjoying it!

It may take you a few weeks to adjust to the lack of sugar and processed foods in your diet. Give yourself time to get used to going without these foods, and in the process, feel free to fill up on all of the Paleo-approved foods, including sweets and burgers, that you *can* eat. After just a week or two, your body will stop requesting high-sugar snacks by hitting you with sugar cravings, and you'll soon find that you enjoy homemade burgers and Paleo-friendly pizza more than the fast-food varieties.

Enjoy these recipes for healthy and delicious Paleo breakfasts, and start experimenting with substitutions that can make your family favorites more Paleo-friendly. Eating Paleo is a tasty adventure, so remember to have fun as you adopt a healthier diet.

GLOSSARY

Celiac disease – a condition in which gluten causes damage to the microvilli of the intestinal tract. Because the microvilli are responsible for absorbing nutrients from foods, people with celiac disease eventually end up becoming malnourished if the condition is left untreated.

Coconut flour – made from finely ground dried coconut. This is a lighter flour than many other nut flours and has little to no "coconut" flavor when used in baking. Available in health food stores and in the organic aisle of many major supermarkets.

Coconut oil – made from pressing the meat of ripe coconut, this oil contains healthy saturated fats. Coconut oil is naturally solid at room temperature or cooler, and it melts into liquid form. It can be stored at room temperature.

Compote – a warm fruit dish made of fruit stewed in its own juices and frequently sweetened with honey or other sweeteners.

Gluten – a protein compound found in cereal grains that is responsible for the elasticity of dough. It is also used in many condiments and packaged foods as a stabilizer.

Gluten-sensitivity – not a diagnosed disease like celiac, but a separate and recognized sensitivity to gluten. The intestinal microvilli are not affected, but people with gluten intolerance or gluten-sensitivity often suffer from bloating, gas, cramping, diarrhea, and other digestive problems.

Grass-fed meats – livestock—including beef, lamb, pork, and game meats—that have been raised in pasture. Frequently also organic and hormone-free, but it's wise to check with the vendor and read the label carefully to be sure. Grass-fed meats have been shown to be higher in healthy fats, such as omega-3 fatty acids, and lower in the unhealthy types of saturated fats.

Hazelnut flour – made from finely ground hazelnuts. It has a slightly sweet flavor that lends itself well to baking and sweet treats, and it's readily available in health food stores or in the organic aisle of many supermarkets.

Insulin – a hormone produced by the body to transport glucose (the form in which our body uses sugar as energy) through the cell membranes to be burned as fuel.

Insulin resistance – a condition in which the body's tissues become less responsive to the release of insulin. This is most often attributed to excess visceral (surrounding the organs) fat caused by poor diet and lack of exercise. Insulin resistance leads to too much glucose being left in the bloodstream (high blood sugar) and often is a precursor to type 2 diabetes.

Legumes – plant foods from the bean family. These include not only beans but English peas, split peas, lentils, and peanuts.

Light olive oil – oil from the second pressing of the olives. The "light" refers to the flavor, rather than the fat content. Light olive oil is best used in baking and in foods when a stronger flavor is undesirable.

Metabolic syndrome – a group of conditions and symptoms that are considered precursors or markers for a future diagnosis of type 2 diabetes. These conditions and symptoms include obesity, excess visceral fat, reduced sensitivity to insulin, and high blood sugar.

Omega-3 fats or fatty acids – one of the essential fats that we need in order to function but that our body do not produce on its own. Omega-3 fats are found in nuts, seeds, olives and their oil, fatty cold-water fish, and grass-fed livestock.

Organic – organic meats and poultry are free of hormones or antibiotics and the animals have been fed a diet of organically grown feed. Organic plant foods are grown without herbicides or pesticides.

Paleo or Paleolithic – referring to the age of humanity that began roughly 2.6 million years ago and lasted until the agricultural age, about ten thousand years ago.

Type 2 diabetes – a form of diabetes that is developed, rather than present at birth. It is often attributed to a lack of exercise and a poor diet, especially a diet high in processed foods, refined flour, sugar, and unhealthy fats.

Voegtlin – gastroenterologist Walter L. Voegtlin, credited with publishing the first version of the Paleolithic, or Paleo, diet in the mid-1970s (*The Stone Age Diet: Based on In-Depth Studies of Human Ecology and the Diet of Man.* New York: Vantage Press, 1975).